"This addition to the literature on healing through the arts is a most welcome contribution. Susan Ridley has done an excellent job of gathering contributors from around the globe who help the reader learn about the use of masks to heal through a fascinating variety of lenses. Such a diverse group of authors, working in many different countries and cultures, make this book intriguing, lively, and a rich read."

Judith A. Rubin, PhD, ATR-BC, *art therapist, psychologist, psychoanalyst, and past president and honorary life member of the American Art Therapy Association*

"Both beginning and experienced therapists and anyone working in arts and health who work with diverse populations and in a variety of settings will find this book extremely informative and applicable. If you are an educator, therapist, or arts and health provider looking for innovative and effective ways to integrate masks into your work, training, or curriculum this book is for you."

Mitchell Kossak, PhD, LMHC, REAT, *professor and coordinator of Counseling and Expressive Arts Therapy at Lesley University*

"This book is an outstanding collection of essays on the usage of masks across disciplines and describes ways in which mask making contributes towards the understanding of the human condition. Susan Ridley's excellent choice of sections, themes, and topics takes us on a journey across the full spectrum of humanity, human relations, and human transformation. This book will hopefully become a requirement for anyone working and studying in a cross-section of fields, from philosophy and religion to psychology, sociology, and human development."

Phillip Speiser, PhD, RDT-BC, *co-founder of International Expressive Arts Therapy Association (IEATA)*

T0372878

The Expressive Use of Masks Across Cultures and Healing Arts

The Expressive Use of Masks Across Cultures and Healing Arts explores the interplay between masks and culture and their therapeutic use in the healing arts such as music, art, dance/movement, drama, play, bibliotherapy, and intermodal.

Each section of the book focuses on a different context, including viewing masks through a cultural lens, masks at play, their role in identity formation (persona and alter ego), healing the wounds from negative life experiences, from the protection of medical masks to helping the healing process, and from expressions of grief to celebrating life stories. Additionally, the importance of cultural sensitivity, including the differences between cultural appreciation and appropriation, is explored. Chapters are written by credentialed therapists to provide unique perspectives on the personal and professional use of masks in the treatment of diverse populations in a variety of settings. A range of experiences are explored, from undergraduate and graduate students to early professionals and seasoned therapists.

The reader will be able to adapt and incorporate techniques and directives presented in these chapters. Readers are encouraged to explore their own cultural heritage, to find their authentic voice, as well as learn how to work with clients who have different life experiences.

Susan Ridley, LPC, NCC, ATR-BC, REAT, associate professor of Creative Arts Therapy at West Liberty University, WV, is an artist, educator, and counselor with over 35 years' experience.

The Expressive Use of Masks Across Cultures and Healing Arts

Edited by Susan Ridley

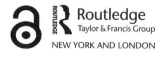

Routledge
Taylor & Francis Group
NEW YORK AND LONDON

First published 2024
by Routledge
605 Third Avenue, New York, NY 10158

and by Routledge
4 Park Square, Milton Park, Abingdon, Oxon, OX14 4RN

Routledge is an imprint of the Taylor & Francis Group, an informa business

ISBN: 9781032430874 (hbk)
ISBN: 9781032430867 (pbk)
ISBN: 9781003365648 (ebk)

DOI: 10.4324/9781003365648

Typeset in Galliard
by Deanta Global Publishing Services, Chennai, India

Contents

Contributors

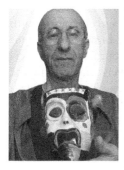

Kamran Afary, PhD, RDT, NT

Kamran is an associate professor of communication studies at California State University Los Angeles and holds a doctorate in performance studies. He is a registered drama therapist (RDT) and a narradrama trainer (NT). He is a published author of several books and articles on narradrama. He is the 2021 recipient of the Teaching Excellence Award by the North American Drama Therapy Association. He created this mask back in 2018 during a narradrama workshop in Lucerne. The workshop focused on intersectionality in the therapeutic encounter, a topic he had the privilege of teaching. Through this vibrant display of pride colors, the aim was to capture the intricate interplay between his previously suppressed identities, such as nationality, ethnicity, queer sexuality, and nonbinary gender. The mask represents the fluidity and interruptions inherent in these aspects of identity, celebrating their unique expressions.

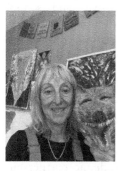

Pat B. Allen, PhD, ATR, IILM

Pat is an author, artist, and art therapist. Her books – *Art Is a Way of Knowing* (1995) and *Art Is a Spiritual Path* (2005) – explore the borders between art, psychology, spirituality, and social action. Her current work, collaborative inquiry through art, which grew out of the open studio process, a way of working she co-created, expands her experiential work to engage jointly held intention for research into social and cultural issues. Pat's novel, *Cronation* (2016), reimagines how her work came into being. She is a core faculty member of the Jewish Studio Project in Berkeley, CA. Her guiding image has always been a coyote. This mask was made to invite that trickster power to always be present in Pat's life and work.

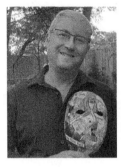

Craig Balfany, ATR-BC, LPC

Craig is a registered and board-certified art therapist (ATR-BC) and licensed professional counselor (LPC). He received his Master of Professional Studies in Art Therapy and Creativity Development from Pratt Institute and additional psychodynamic training through the Institute for Expressive Analysis in New York. His clinical and educational experience spans over 30 years. His art therapy practice has engaged children, adolescents, and adults who have experienced trauma that often resulted in mental, physical, and chemical health issues. He integrates individual psychology and humanistic and existential theories into his holistic and socially interested approach to art therapy practice, training, and supervision. He is actively engaged in the creative process that values exploring metaphors, encouraging expression, and building social connectedness. His creative identity is rooted in ceramics, sculpture, photography, gardening, and mask making. He has presented papers, panel discussions, and conducted workshops on art therapy at professional conferences as well as to local educational, mental health, and arts organizations.

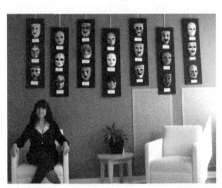

Lucy Barbera, PhD, LCAT

Lucy is a New York State-licensed creative arts therapist whose clinical work spans medical, psychiatric, and special education settings, as a medical art therapist, special education principal, and school district administrator. From 1996–2019, she served on the faculty of the Humanistic Multicultural Education Graduate program at SUNY New Paltz, developing and teaching undergraduate and graduate courses in expressive arts therapy and expressive arts and social justice leadership. She facilitates professional development training and lectures widely on trauma-informed creative arts therapy and the power of the arts to build resilience and mitigate the negative effects of trauma. Currently, she is facilitating trauma-informed programs in academic partnership with the University at Albany's School of Social Welfare. She maintains a private practice, using a trauma-informed model, working with self-harming/suicidal teens, children, and adults with life-threatening medical conditions, addiction, and complex trauma.

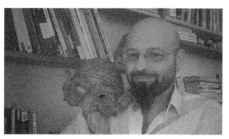

Dov Blum-Yazdi, PhD

Dov is a certified drama therapist, a registered senior supervisor, a clinical criminologist, a graduate of the psychotherapy body-mind-spirit program, and a postdoctoral student at the Laboratory of Psychology and Special Education, University of Crete. Dov is a lecturer at the School of Creative Arts Therapies, University of Haifa, Israel, and the director of the MA program ultra-orthodox track at Haifa University. He is the founder of The Leelah Play. His main research interests are in the areas connecting research and clinical work, focusing mainly on play, drama, and its connection to psychoanalytic theories. Dov has extensive clinical experience as a drama therapist in private and public practice; he has a specialist position in group therapy at the Ministry of Education. The mask for Dov is an avatar; an embodiment of an alter-ego in a client.

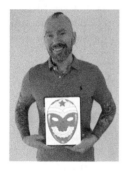

Michael Boyce, MA, LPCC, ATR

Michael was born in Ohio and worked as a caricature artist at the local amusement parks. They were such a hit in their first summer drawing funny pictures of guests at the amusement parks. In California, they established themself as artists and ran a comic book store. Michael furthered their education by going to art school in San Francisco and then created and published two children's books explaining the difficult subject of living without a home. Michael combined all their strengths in art, comics, and helping and then went on to earn a master's degree in counseling and art therapy. Michael is a licensed professional clinical counselor and a registered art therapist. Michael is a person-centered therapist and adheres to Carl Roger's School of Therapy. Michael's superpower is to spread empathy, compassion, and understanding to everyone.

René A. Burgoyne, ATRL-BC, LPC

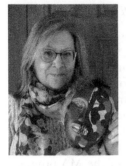

René is an art therapist and disabled Army veteran. She has studied to become a level-one trauma therapist through the Expressive Arts Therapy Institute. She has presented at the 46th Annual American Art Therapy Conference on *Hoarding Disorder: The Monster that Lies Within*, and most recently at the 53rd Annual Conference panel presentation, *Bridging the Gap: Providing a Non-Verbal Means to Understanding Non-Art Therapy Modalities.* She has been working with service members and veterans for over 20 years. She is passionate about helping fellow service members/veterans transition back into civilian life. The mask she created symbolizes the duality of who she represents. One part of her is a veteran with wounds that continue to heal. It's difficult to see the wounds which are appropriate to the current work setting. The other part is the creative arts therapist. She brings a bright, colorful perspective to an otherwise difficult setting. The violet combines the calm stability of blue and the fierce energy of red, providing what is needed for each art therapy session. The feathers and other shiny objects are for protection and to reflect the necessary elements back to the veterans.

Nancy Jo Cardillo, PhD, BC-DMT, LMHC

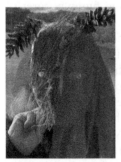

Nancy is coordinator and core faculty for undergraduate art and expressive art therapies (AT/EAT) majors and dual-degree students at Lesley University. She has taught courses at the graduate and undergraduate level on integrated arts in education and therapy nationally, internationally, and on the Cambridge campus. Students have traveled with her to Haiti and South Africa to engage in service, learning and arts in the community. In Nancy Jo's professional practice, she regularly supervises interns and alumni and conducts dance/movement therapy (DMT) groups for a diverse range of individuals across the lifespan. Areas of interest include the intersection of kinesthetic empathy and body image in DMT/EAT and embodied culture and conflict in pedagogy and practice. Nancy Jo's mask was prompted by a line in one of Laurel Doggett's poems about a bull who appears with no warning, blocking the view and stubbornly refusing to move. When confronted in a bullying way, the mask instils courage to charge and take charge.

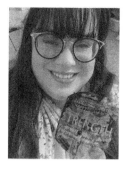

Jane Carriere MAAT, ATR-P

Jane is a recent graduate of Saint Mary-of-the-Woods College. She has served at Advocate Aurora Health in medical art therapy for the past three years. During the strain of the COVID-19 pandemic, Jane prepared and studied for providing art therapy through virtual sessions that helped manage the pandemic-based shifts from in-person open studio groups to online working studio groups. Jane did her school-based internships at Advocate Aurora Health and currently serves as an extern art therapist, managing the still-online factions of the open art therapy studio processes.

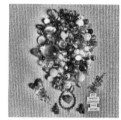

Krystal L. Demaine, PhD, REAT, MT-BC, RYT

Krystal is a professor of expressive therapies in the School of Visual and Performing Arts at Endicott College in Beverly, MA, USA, and is the author of *The Roots and Rhythm of the Heart*, which shares her journey through grief, music, and heartful healing. Her approach to teaching and therapy is grounded in science, play, creativity, and imagination. The mask assemblage is built of several small and large round glass marbles inherited in part by the author's grandmother and shaped into the author's face. The marbles are light in color and not opaque. The lower part of the face is cupped by symbols of care and comfort including a red heart stone at the center, which is surrounded by a Star of David bracelet and two adjacent brass Buddha statues, all offering symbols of protection and grounding spiritual beliefs. Scented lavender flowers are sprinkled around the lower sides and to the right are the words "play", "medicine", "understand", "trust", and "journey." The reflection and refraction of light onto the glass marbles allows light to pass through and also mirror its viewer.

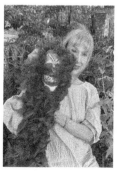

Pam Dunne PhD, RDT/BCT, NT

Pam is a clinical psychologist, registered drama therapist/board-certified trainer (RDT/BCT), narradrama trainer, and professor emerita at California State University, Los Angeles. She is a published author, with over a dozen books, films, articles, and book chapters and awards for her contribution to the field of drama therapy. Pam is the director of the Drama Therapy Institute of Los Angeles (DTILA) and the Creative Therapies Center (CTC). She conducts training and workshops internationally. Pam is the former president of the North American Drama Therapy Association (NADTA) and a founding member of its Board of Examiners. As Pam peers out from behind the mask, she is struck by the invitation to play and run freely in a natural setting. She also connects with the softness and long purple flowing hair of the mask, which invites her into the gentleness and kindness expressed by this mask and the free spirit. She also senses the healing transformational power of the mask, which she connects to her recovery from an overpowering illness. She feels a lightness and her breath returning, as she flows with the mask and breathes in these healing properties.

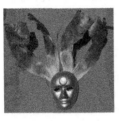

Tamar Reva Einstein, PhD, REAT

Tamar is an expressive arts therapist, artist, and researcher. Since 1987, she has crossed cultural borders in Jerusalem with the arts as her compass and guide. Tamar continues to work and live in Jerusalem and is interested in the cultural richness and imagery of this unique city. Art as a mother tongue is her guiding message in her clinical and academic life. Mask making has been a meaningful part of the student training, clinical, and personal work she has done over the years.

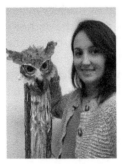

Terri Giller-Etheridge, M.Ed., ATR-BC, LPC

Terri is the instructor of Creative Arts Therapy at West Liberty University in West Virginia and owns a private practice, Calling Cadence Counseling and Art Therapy Services, LLC. Terri earned her Master of Education in Counseling/Art Therapy from the University of Louisville in 2007 and has worked as an art therapist since then, working with a variety of client populations. Terri began teaching at WLU in 2021 and enjoys the balance of teaching, providing therapy services, and tending to her own artist self. The mask in the photo was created in response to exploring her roles and aspirations as an educator, teacher, and counselor – representing "the sage" archetype. Terri hopes to embody the sage archetype by continually gathering information, acquiring knowledge, and always pursuing truth. This mask was inspired by Terri's love of bird imagery and is made using some of the fabric she created by dyeing with foraged acorns and walnuts.

Jhan Groom, MACP, RCAT

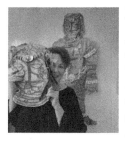

Jhan Groom, MACP, is a registered psychologist and a registered Canadian art therapist in Calgary, Alberta, Canada who has been in practice for over 17 years. Mask work has always been a part of her practice, and she has taught mask workshops at schools and national art therapy conferences. Jhan has studied masks, mask history, and mask psychology extensively. Of particular interest is how masks reveal, rather than conceal, aspects of the individual, which led to the protocol documented in this book. Shown with Jhan is the mask of an ancient wise woman and guide she discovered within herself during a workshop. Along the bottom of the mask it says, "Old woman, rooted, grounded by her body weight, contains the whole universe."

Erin Hein MS, LPC, ATR-BC

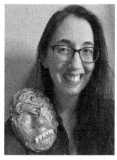

Erin serves as an art therapist at Advocate Aurora Health, and as an art therapist leader at Donna Lexa Art Centers. Erin has been an art therapist with Donna Lexa since 2010 and has been a medical art therapist since 2014. Her practice specialties include cancer care, grief navigation, supporting persons with disability with creativity and imagination, and psychotherapy for mental health. Her philosophical approach to art therapy is from an existential perspective, enhanced by Jungian principles. One of Erin's favorite pastimes in art therapy is bringing the arts and art therapy to Advocate Aurora staff, encouraging self-care and self-exploration or growth.

Lisa D. Hinz, PhD, ATR-BC

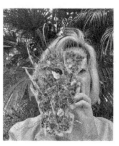

Lisa is a licensed clinical psychologist and a registered, board-certified art therapist in the United States. She is an associate professor of art therapy psychology at Dominican University of California and the director of the doctoral program in art therapy psychology. Dr Hinz is the author of many published works in the field of art therapy, including the second edition of her book, *Expressive Therapies Continuum: A Framework for the Use of Art in Therapy*. She maintains a private practice focused on eating and wellness issues. Her mask is a hopeful talisman, imbued with the power to aid her in the transition from mother to crone. She is somewhere in the middle of leaving motherhood and not yet embracing crone. When she looks in the mirror each day to brush her teeth or comb her hair, she is surprised by the appearance of the crone and wants to erase her, or at least erase the lines that define her. She would rather instead welcome and embrace her. This mask is a first attempt to welcome the crone.

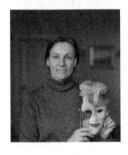

Ksenia Ilinskaya, Md, NT

Ksenia received her master's degree in psychology and a diploma in systemic family therapy. She has been working with families since 2002. She is a professor in the master's program of systemic family therapy at HSE University (Higher School of Economics), Moscow, a narradrama trainer (NT), and a translator in Russian of articles in the narradrama field. Utilizing drama therapy and the creative arts in both her teaching and in therapeutic work with clients, Ksenia's pioneering work in narradrama in Russia includes running workshops, conferences, and training for professionals and educators. Her "Mask of My Future Self" incorporates various colors to make it vibrant and unique. She feels that her mask has something to communicate with the people around her, which was quite surprising. Several years have passed since she engaged in projects, collaborating with groups, families, and individuals. Now, she is presenting herself alongside her colleagues. It seems that she truly has something significant to express. Isn't it magical, the act of creating a mask?

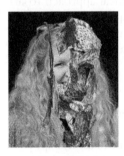

Jill McNutt PhD, LPC, ATR-BC, ATRL, ATCS

Jill serves as an art therapist at Advocate Aurora Health, Director of Graduate Art Therapy at Edgewood College, and director of administration at the Art Therapy House, Inc. She has been a medical art therapist since 2002, and an art therapy educator since 2012. Her practice specialties include art therapy in cancer care and epilepsy, art therapy education, employee/staff wellness, and facilitation of open studio processes. Her philosophical approach to art therapy is through a feminist lens with attributes from narrative and psychodynamic perspectives. Jill's most valued art therapy venues are group facilitation and working with patients facing life-challenging situations.

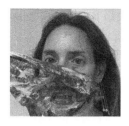

Einat Metzl, PhD, LMFT, ATR-BC, APT

Einat is an art therapy professor and the chair of the graduate art therapy program at Bar Ilan University, Israel. She received her clinical training at Loyola Marymount University's graduate department of MFT with specialized training in art therapy, where she had also taught and chaired the program after completing her doctoral degree at Florida State University. Metzl's research focus includes how creativity supports wellbeing, recovery after natural disasters, post-war and grief support, early intervention work, and understanding the use of art within different groups and settings. She chose to create her mask from a simple Saran Wrap most of us have at home. Applying the paint there meant brush strokes were very close to her skin; she could feel them precisely, yet they did not touch her. The colors, textures, and spaces carry meanings for her. She took an image while taking the mask halfway off, revealing both truths – as how she is seen and as intentionally presented. The moments of intentionally taking off or putting on aspects of ourselves are precious moments of vulnerable reveal.

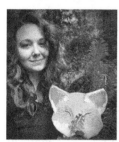

Charlene K. Michener, MA, ATR, CTP

Charlene works as an outpatient drug and alcohol counselor and art therapist for individual and group settings. Charlene utilizes art therapy in these settings to assist the traditional recovery programming as an opportunity to learn through action and reflection, while also working on impacts of environments, families, and other co-occurring mental health struggles. Charlene believes that, through the creative process and use of metaphors, individuals can learn about emotional regulation, relearn self-identity without addiction, and pave a golden road for recovery. Charlene has an extensive background in ceramic art, but also enjoys working with photography and wooden or natural mediums. When Charlene has time to create art for herself, she typically creates ceramic masks or anything surrounding the theme of nature, especially foxes and acorns. The photographed mask with Charlene represents her personal and professional growth with the desire to inspire hope within her clients. The fox represents the self, while the oak leaf is hope. Hope is like acorns; plant them well, tend them carefully, and they will grow to be as mighty as the oak.

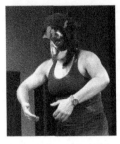

Gina Holloway Mulder, MA, VMTR, PGDA

Gina Holloway Mulder has worked with various populations creatively and therapeutically through voice- and movement work since 1999, incorporating voice movement therapy (VMT) into her practice in 2007, when she qualified as South Africa's first VMT. Gina runs a private practice, regularly lectures in tertiary institutions in South Africa, and actively contributes to the global growth of VMT by running workshops and assisting VMT practitioner training both in SA and abroad. She has served multiple terms on the International Association of Voice Movement Therapy (IAVMT) board of directors and has written and edited for the *Practitioners of VMT Journal*. She recently co-edited the book *Singing the Psyche: Uniting Thought and Feeling Through Voice: Voice Movement Therapy in Practice*. The "Great Bird Mother" mask represents her inner wisdom and intuition. The Bird Mother brings forth her strength and energy and connects her to the ancestors and to the shamanic healer in her. The Bird Mother sees, she holds, she nurtures, and protects. She links the heavens and the earth, bridging the natural world with the supernatural realm. The Great Bird Mother mask sits in Gina's studio as a constant reminder of her inner resources and resilience, as well as her greater purpose.

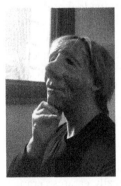

Shiu Hei Larry Ng, MPhil, MA, RDT, NADTA

Larry Ng is a registered drama therapist and a certified Feldenkrais Method® practitioner. He has also completed professional diploma training in Satir transformational systemic therapy (Level 2), and in neuro-dramatic-play (Advanced Diploma) under Dr Sue Jennings and is now in training in the therapeutic spiral model of psychodrama. As an artist, he was trained in physical and devising theater (Lecoq approach) and corporeal mime (Decroux system) and specializes in mask making. He learned mask design and making from Donato Sartori, Matteo Destro, and Renzo Sindoca. He is also a playback theater practitioner who has completed all four levels of training, with more than ten years of ongoing experience of practice. He has also been working through different kinds of applied theater modalities to serve a wide range of the population in the community. He was also academically trained in philosophy (BA, first-class honors and Master of Philosophy degree) and drama education (master's degree). The mask represents thinking, "I think a lot...and I need to think, as humans are so complicated and there are too many injustices in society… But what else is needed besides thinking?"

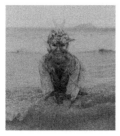

Angie Richardson, ATCL, DipTchg, BEd, MAAT (Clinical), HCPC UK

Angie is a child of the storm, an experienced, clinically registered creative arts therapist and registered teacher from Aotearoa, New Zealand. Through her private practice, Creative Harmony, she has worked with children/teens/adults and families using a multi-modal approach. She has contracted her therapeutic services to schools and organizations and provided supervision for clinical students and therapists. Her therapeutic modalities include drama/play therapy, creative visual arts, sandtray, sounding, and movement. A passion for dramatic play stems from having run a drama school for children, years of freeform improvisation training and play sessions, along with profound personal healing from this modality. She is passionate about advocating for playFULLness in schools to support *tamariki*/children with their wellbeing and learning, including those who have experienced trauma. Angie has a chapter on hut making included in an international dramatherapy book and an article published on mask making during COVID-19. She has facilitated numerous workshops and has lectured in the MA in Creative Arts Therapy degree program at Whitecliffe in Auckland. Underpinning her practice is an acknowledgment of the urgent call for connection to Gaia and a belief in the alchemy of the expressive arts to empower people to find their soul medicine.

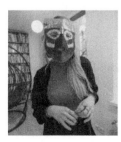

Nathalie Robelot-Timtchenko, MA-ET

Nathalie holds a master's degree in clinical mental health counseling with a specialization in intermodal expressive arts therapy from Lesley University in Cambridge. She is a professional member of the International Expressive Arts Therapy Association (IEATA) and the European Federation of Art Therapy (EFAT). While most of her life was spent cross-culturally, eight years were in Kyiv, Ukraine, up until 2021. Ukraine is home for Nathalie. Nathalie has over a decade of clinical experience working with groups, individuals, and families within a variety of settings as well as cultures. Nathalie's expertise is in working with individuals facing challenges related to self-worth, acculturation, displacement, complex trauma, crisis, suicidal ideation, depression, anxiety, family conflict, and interpersonal difficulties. Nathalie founded and directs First Aid of the Soul, which offers free psychosocial and emotional support services to those being affected by Russia's war against Ukraine. This mask represents the fight for freedom of the Ukrainian people and the unbreakable resilience of the nation. It has been truly heartbreaking and immensely painful to witness the current atrocities taking place in and against Ukraine. This mask is a symbol of power, unbreakable strength, and hope for a victorious tomorrow.

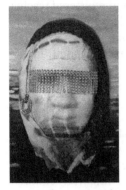

Susan Ridley, PhD, LPC, NCC, REAT, ATR-BC

Susan is an associate professor of creative arts therapy at West Liberty University and chair of the Department of Art Therapy and Counseling. She is a licensed professional counselor (LPC), a nationally certified counselor (NCC), a registered expressive arts therapist (REAT), and a board-certified art therapist (ATR-BC). She is an artist, educator, and counselor with over 35 years' experience working with diverse communities of various ages, abilities, and disabilities. She believes in the therapeutic power of creative expression to heal, empower, and transform. As a Celtic artist, she is inspired by nature and specializes in landscapes, seascapes, and animals. She is passionate about community art projects and painting murals that bring people together in positive self-expression. Her research interest is in identity, using mirrors as a tool for self-reflection, self-care, and arts-based research. Her mask represents "seen and not heard," a mantra she grew up with as a child. Unfortunately, not much has changed, as women's rights continue to be eroded, control over body autonomy is reduced, and the march towards women's equality is forgotten.

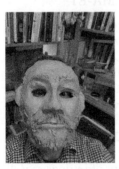

Binyamin Rose, MSc

Binyamin is completing doctoral studies with the gender studies department at Bar-Ilan University, Israel on gender and sexual diversity in contemporary Jungian psychoanalytic practice. Rose is also an artist, psychiatric social worker, and supervising Jungian analyst. Having studied in the UK at Oxford, Manchester and London, Rose has worked with LGBTQIA+ people since 1998 in both community and hospital settings. Rose moved to Jerusalem in 2006, and, while managing an HIV testing clinic, established the therapy service at the Jerusalem Open House for Pride and Tolerance in 2012. Since completing training with the Institute for Jungian Psychology in honor of Erich Neumann, Rose continues to supervise clinical social work at the Open House and works in private practice in Jerusalem.

Natallia Sakovich, MA

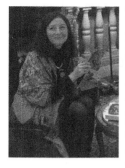

Natallia has been practicing art therapy since 1998. Her graduate thesis at the Tashkent State Institute of Culture was about the influence of human factors on the roles we choose. Moreover, dance, arts, and photography have always been a part of her life, influencing her state by helping her to survive, respond, or calm down. Her degree in psychology (Postgraduate Academy) enabled her to make a tight linkage between those two directions. In 1998, she joined Alexander Kopytin's art therapy training course (Saint Petersburg). It was the first post-soviet enrollment of art therapists. She completed the course and got the diploma of art therapy. She joined the Art Therapy Association (Russia) and started practicing sand therapy. In 2000–2002, she took June Atherton's sand therapy course at the Irish Sand Therapy Institute. She has developed training courses in art and sand therapy and provided training for over 2,000 experts in Belarus and is the author of 19 books and guidance. Her numerous articles have been published in professional and non-specialized magazines. She hosted TV programs and participated in various shows and is the leading expert in art and sand therapy in Belarus. She also teaches art therapy at the Family Development School.

Nancy S. Scherlong, LCSW, SEP, CJT/PTR, CM

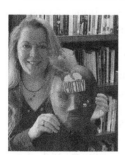

Nancy is the owner of Change Your Narrative LCSW PLLC and is trained in EMDR, SE, IFS, MBSR, DBT, poetry, journal therapy, and psychodrama. She is currently the president of the International Federation for Biblio-Poetry Therapy (IFBPT) and a long-time member of the National Association for Poetry Therapy (NAPT). She is a senior adjunct faculty for Adelphi University's online and residential MSW programs and has created a certificate program for applied expressive arts in counseling. She is core faculty at the Therapeutic Writing Institute and teaches at the Kint Institute in their foundation year for trauma-focused expressive arts. She is a published author and poet. This mask is, in fact, a metaphor for the past several years. There has been so much richness and mind-expansion in her work, yet so much struggle in the world and in many people's daily lives. On a personal level, four years ago, she lost her mother, who was, for most of her early life, her best friend and companion in reading literature (and in reading every academic assignment she ever wrote!). Just two years later, she lost her sister-in-law to a merciless cancer, so there were lots of red eyes for a while. Through everything, poetry has been her sustenance and support, in addition to family and being able to count on her own multilayered self.

Maru Serricchio-Joiner, PhD, LMFT, ATR-BC

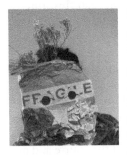

Maru is an art therapy professor at Loyola Marymount University in Los Angeles, CA. Her research is on grief responses and support in the workplace within Mexican culture. She continues to be an active practitioner and artist, working with individuals, families, and groups from all walks of life and providing workshops regarding ways to transform experiences of loss, grief, and trauma through creative tools. She created her mask from materials that were in her home as resources for building, wrapping, and even containing. As a therapist, working with grief and loss, trauma, and transformation and acceptance of identity, resources are crucial to thriving. She found herself using the "fragile" tape to put together the mask and go across where the eyes would be, to signify the fragility of the moment and to highlight the importance of storytelling as our own power; we get to see and tell/re-author our story as it makes sense and relates to us. Lastly, there is a softness to the mask, using tissue paper, to embody the many gifts life has to offer. These resources are some of the many that she hopes to use to guide her clients, students, and supervisees in their journey.

Tsufit Shemer, MA Dramatherapy

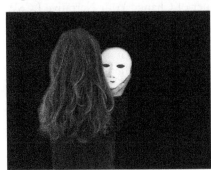

Tsufit is a drama therapist and a community theater director. She works with children and adolescents with special needs as a drama therapist and directs community theater with groups of seniors and doctoral students in The Program for Hermeneutics and Cultural Studies at Bar-Ilan University, Israel. Her research interests include old age performances in contemporary theater. She lives and works in Israel. The mask is the essence of drama therapy, a unique prop that is a magic paradox of dynamic and static, hidden and discovered, familiar and foreign, ancient, and transformative.

Hannah Sherebrin, ATR-BC, OATR, YAHAT

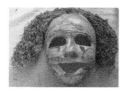

Hannah is an art therapist specializing in trauma, bereavement, losses, and depression with adult and senior populations. She provides palliative care in home hospice situations for her clients. She trained in Canada, but lives part of the year in Israel. She supervises professionals and maintains a small private practice. She offers art therapy bereavement support groups for complex grief. She has published numerous articles and book chapters, and has presented workshops and lectures, including a keynote at international conferences in Canada, the US, Europe, Israel, and South America. Currently, she is the most-recent vice-president of the Israeli arts therapy association (YAHAT), and the registration and supervision chair of the Ontario Art Therapy Association. Hannah is a passionate photographer and potter and has presented photographs, drawings, and pottery in a number of exhibitions. She is 80 years young and forever growing through touching trauma in others and herself.

Todd Wharton, MA, CRPO, OATR, CPT

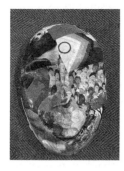

Todd Wharton has been working with children, youth, and young adults in a career spanning over 40 years. He is a registered psychotherapist (CRPO), registered art therapist (OATR), and certified play therapist (CPT) who is working in a publicly funded tertiary care children's hospital and private practice and previously at a provincially-run children and youth mental health and developmental services center. His scope of practice has incorporated numerous people with a wide range of medical and mental health diagnoses, many who have been followed for years. Through interactions in various settings, Todd has been able to integrate his educational knowledge with experience to develop a collaborative philosophy and approach that has proven effective in assisting others with addressing their concerns. Currently, the focus has been on developing an understanding and skill set for working with gender-diverse individuals. This mask was created using collage and represents various aspects of who he is, including his professional and personal life. It was created especially for this book to give the reader a peek at who the author of this chapter is.

Acknowledgments

We stand on the shoulders of all those who came before us. The pioneers who laid the foundations for us to practice expressive arts therapy in its many forms across the world. The theorists whose frameworks guide our work with vulnerable populations. The champions and advocates who promote the therapeutic arts, and the family and friends who support us in our endeavors. I would also like to thank our teachers and supervisors who pass on their knowledge and experience to the next generation. And thank you to the multitude of therapists working on the front lines who toil day-in and day-out to make the world a better place for all of us. A special thank you goes to the contributors willing to share their experiences working in different countries, in diverse therapeutic practices and modalities. Each one shares their insights and personal experiences, passing the torch to the next generation of students and therapists.

Thank you to Routledge: Taylor & Francis Group for giving me the opportunity to bring this book to fruition. A special thank you goes to Amanda Savage, Editor – Mental Health, and Ellie Broadhurst, Editorial Assistant for all your hard work and expertise. And to the production staff for bringing this book to life. Without your help, none of this would be possible.

Introduction

Masks have been used by many cultures across the centuries for multiple purposes – in religious practices and ceremonial dances, during warfare, as entertainment, in criminal activities, and as a tool for healing. Masks are steeped in cultural heritage and rooted in historical context. It is important to distinguish between cultural appreciation and cultural appropriation when working with masks, since the lines are sometimes blurred and it is easy to step unwittingly into the gray area. Cultural appreciation, as the name implies, appreciates another culture and broadens one's perspective. Immersing yourself in other cultures is a great way to better understand the people you work with, your similarities and differences, and to broaden your understanding of different ways of living (Howie et al., 2013). Cultural appreciation involves honoring the history of the people, places, and things. For example, joining in the celebration of a cultural or spiritual event by wearing appropriate clothing is cultural appreciation. This assumes that you have been invited to the cultural or spiritual event and have asked your hosts what is most appropriate to wear.

Ziff and Rao (1997) described cultural appropriation as taking ownership of cultural artifacts and intellectual property that are not your own, without acknowledgment or permission, and using it out of context from its spiritual or cultural roots. Lalonde (2019) found three factors that make up cultural appropriation: not recognizing or ignoring claims to property belonging to the marginalized group, deliberately misidentifying a particular group and perpetuating stereotypes that are harmful to them, and benefiting from the exploitation of others. For example, selling tribal insignia without permission to benefit yourself or wearing stereotypical ethnic clothing that demeans the culture and its people. Cattien and Stopford (2022) suggest that we make a critical appraisal of our sociohistorical and cultural relationship with other cultures to determine if it's appreciation or appropriation, bearing in mind who has power and privilege in these choices.

DOI: 10.4324/9781003365648-1

Masks hold a fascination for many people because of their historical meaning, religious/spiritual significance, performative versatility, and therapeutic qualities. Since masks and mask making cross cultural barriers and there are commonalities in materials and techniques, it is suggested that the reader explore the historical origins of the mask specific to the culture of the people you work with (e.g., colors, shape, materials, usage, etc.). By exploring the context of the masks within the culture of the client, the reader can help them to delve deeper into ancestral roots and identity. This will help to ground them in their cultural heritage and help them to authentically express their identity and how they choose to identify.

The Structure of This Book

This book explores the interplay between masks and culture and their therapeutic use in the healing arts across various expressive therapies: art, music, movement/dance, drama, play, bibliotherapy, and intermodal. Chapters have been written by credentialed therapists to provide unique perspectives on the personal and professional use of masks in the treatment of diverse populations. It is divided into six parts, with each section focused on a particular theme. Part I reviews the historical use of masks in religious, spiritual, and cultural practices and how they are used in modern times within this context. In Chapter 1, Susan Ridley explores the rites, rituals, and transformation of masks. In Chapter 2, Nancy Scherlong writes about the multitudes and parts of the self through poetry and bibliotherapy. Chapter 3, Dov Blum-Yazdi explores the Leelah Play and the use of avatars in trauma-informed dramatherapy. In Chapter 4, Shiu Hei Larry Ng reviews the transformative journey of mask in drama therapy and suggests reversing the sequence in Lecoq's physical theater pedagogy. In Chapter 5, Gina Holloway Mulder shares her work integrating voice movement therapy and mask work in South Africa.

Part II focuses on the use of masks in the context of play, particularly with children, adolescents, and young adults with various abilities/disabilities. In Chapter 6, Angie Richardson shares her experiences cultivating imagination and the expression of playFULLness with indigenous boys in New Zealand. In Chapter 7, Jhan Groom writes about mask work and increasing imagination and developing self-awareness in children. She believes that through a false face one finds a true face. In Chapter 8, Tsufit Shemer shares her experience of using neutral masks with young adolescents attending group drama therapy sessions in middle school in Israel. Nancy Jo Cardillo explores the use of masks to encourage victim empathy in teenage girls in the criminal justice system in Chapter 9.

Part III focuses on the use of masks in identity formation, persona, and alter ego, and as a metaphor. In Chapter 10, Craig Balfany uses metaphors to explore personal and professional identities. In Chapter 11, Tamar Reva Einstein shares the process of making masks with her phototherapy students in East and West Jerusalem. In Chapter 12, Krystal Demaine describes the experiences undergraduate expressive therapy students encounter with the mask as they engage in ritual, dialogue, and reflection. In Chapter 13, Pam Dunne, Kamran Afary, and Ksenia Ilinskaya describe their work with masks in narradrama. In Chapter 14, Binyamin Rose shares his experience of mask making to explore gender and sexuality identity.

Part IV includes the healing properties of masks and mask making with those who have experienced trauma, abuse, violence, and war (i.e., active military, veterans, civilians). In Chapter 15, Michael Boyce shares their experiences of using a superhero persona to overcome negative life experiences. Chapter 16 describes the work of Maru Serricchio-Joiner and Einat S. Metzl with veterans transitioning to civilian life. Chapter 17, René A. Burgoyne writes about her work in an art therapy open studio healing the wounds of war as veterans return home from combat. Chapter 18, Natalie Rebelot-Timtchenko describes her work with First Aid of The Soul (FAS), which provides free and accessible mental health support to Ukrainians affected by the war with Russia. Chapter 19, Ksenia Ilinskaya, Kamran Afary, and Pam Dunne describe their workshops in Russia working with masks using a trauma-informed narradrama method.

Part V explores the changing use of masks from the protection of medical masks to helping with the healing process. In Chapter 20, Jill McNutt, Erin Hein, and Jane Carriere write about mask making as a featured process in a hospital-based open studio. In Chapter 21, Susan Ridley and Terri Giller-Etheridge report on an interview with an undergraduate student and her father about the transformation of a radiation mask and how it helped them become closer as a family through the adversity of his illness. Chapter 22 explores Lucy Barbera's work with the avatar to foster hope and healing. In Chapter 23, Charlene K. Michener describes the exploration of using a Kintsugi-inspired mask making process in addiction. Chapter 24, Lisa D. Hinz writes about her work using therapeutic masks in the treatment of eating disorders.

Part VI focuses on the expression of grief and celebration of the life of a loved one who has passed. Chapter 25, written by Natallia Sakovich, reviews the use of a crisis sand therapy technique to help a client overcome her grief and loss of her marriage through her husband's infidelity. In Chapter 26, Hannah Sherebrin shares the power of masks in processing grief in a bereavement support group in Israel. In Chapter 27, Todd Wharton shares his work using masks to explore inner emotions in a children's hospital with patients diagnosed with cancer. In Chapter 28, Pat B. Allen explores her personal experience of grief and loss and the implications of using masks in treatment.

It is hoped that this book is informative for both beginning and experienced expressive therapists and that it provides practical applications to your work. All the chapters are a synthesis of the contributors' professional and personal experiences working with diverse populations, utilizing a range of expressive therapy techniques in a variety of settings. The chapters cover a wide range of experiences from undergraduate and graduate students to early professionals and experienced therapists. Each chapter stands on its own merits as well as spans a wide range of disciplines and practices. There may be differences in terminology, since the contributions come from a wide range of cultural experiences and training. These countries include Canada, China, Israel, New Zealand, Russia, South Africa, Ukraine, the United Kingdom, and the United States. As such, the editor has decided to respect linguistic choices and terminology.

References

Cattien, J., & Stopford, R. J. (2022). The appropriating subject: Cultural appreciation, property and entitlement. *Philosophy and Social Criticism*, 1–18. https://journals.sagepub.com/doi/10.1177/01914537211059515

Howie, P., Prasad, S., & Kristel, J. (2013). *Using art therapy with diverse populations: Crossing cultures and abilities.* Jessica Kingsley Publishers.

Lalonde, D. (2019). Does cultural appropriation cause harm? *Politics, Groups, and Identities, 9*(2), 329–346. https://doi.org/10.1080/21565503.2019.1674160

Ziff, B., & Rao, P. V. (1997). *Borrowed power: Essays on cultural appropriation.* Rutgers University Press.

Cultural Masks

Criminal Masks

Chapter 1

Masks

Rites, Rituals, and Transformations

Susan Ridley

From the dawn of time, masks have been integral to the cultural practices of diverse populations across the world. Some of the earliest known drawings of masks date back to the Palaeolithic period in paintings on cave walls in Tassali, Spain, and in Dordogne, France. These figures are depicted wearing a variety of animal masks including a stag's head, an owl's face, wolf ears, a goat's beard, bear paws, and a horse's tail (Sivin, 1986). Anthropologists suggest that this mask imagery represents priests or shamans taking part in a ritual of transformation (Foreman, 2000). Masks seem to possess a mythical-religious presence which bestows the wisdom and power of specific animals or birds onto the wearer (Dunn-Snow & Joy-Smellie, 2000). The oldest known masks, at 9,000 years old, were found in caves in the Judean Hills in Israel (Hershman, 2014). The Neolithic masks features include a round human-like face with empty eye sockets, truncated noses, and gaping mouths. They also had small, pierced holes around the mask, indicating that hair or other adornments could be woven around the face, making them even more realistic. It is thought that these masks may have been used in religious ceremonies, rites, and rituals.

Historically, masks have been used in rituals to bless crops, for fertility, to receive blessings, celebrate festivals and holidays, or to appease the gods. Numerous cultures use masks as part of ceremonial death-related rituals to help the recently deceased to enter the ancestral realm. Masks have also been used to guard their community or to instill terror in the hearts of enemies (Edson, 2009). Masks have also accompanied priests and shamans to the underworld to appease restless spirits or to mediate between the living and the dead (Patterson & Donahue, 2013). Berlejeung and Filitz (2018) believe that masks create a relational connection and a liminal space between worlds: the physical and spiritual, the seen and unseen, and life and death.

The key element of masks is transformation. They help the wearer to move from one role to another or provide the opportunity to try on various identities. The mask is a means of separating the wearer from themselves and creating the "other" persona, shielding their identity, and imbuing them

DOI: 10.4324/9781003365648-3

with power and status. Edson (2009) wrote that "by their unusual nature, they arouse curiosity, stimulate the imagination, and transport the viewer [and the wearer] from the seemingly mundane activities of daily life to a different, often mystical time" (p. 7).

The effects of masks are generally separated into two categories: the impact on the wearer and the impact on those viewing the mask (Roy, 2000). For the wearer, the mask can help them to increase their reflective practice and connect them to their unconscious processes. They can also promote self-reflection and self-knowledge without the pressures of direct self-disclosure (Elliott & Conneller, 2020). The wearer does not need to be vulnerable or frightened of other people's reactions when they embody the persona of the mask they wear (West et al., 2001). For the observer, the mask creates a sense of alienation and separation, allowing them to discover their own meaning from the scene that they witness (Roy, 2016). However, for McNiff (2004), the mask has its own identity, separate from the wearer. This can be seen in the use of avatars and neutral masks where the mask itself is the focus of therapeutic interventions, not the wearer. Non-representational approaches to masks focus on what they do rather than what they depict.

The power of the mask resides in its ability to evoke emotional responses (Harris, 2021). Foreman (2000) identified six ways that masks are used:

- Invoking the "other," such as another person, a demonic spirit, an animal, etc.
- As an object that has been sculpted, modeled, cast, painted, woven, etc.
- Embodied by holding in the hand, worn on the face, attached to the body, etc.
- Used in the practice of magic, ritual, religion, war, decoration, performance, etc.
- To connect the social, individual, or psychological functions of the mask.
- As transformation, dissimulation, mimetic, transference, induce fear, etc.

Landy (1994) identified four ways that a mask could be used in therapeutic practice. These include representing two sides in a conflict or dilemma by externalizing the issue, for example, with an inside-outside mask. Decorating the mask to reveal the polarity of emotions can help clients to integrate disparate thoughts and feelings of how they feel inside versus what they project to others. Clients can also explore their identity by decorating the mask with symbolic representations of the wearer's strengths and values, for example, by choosing an animal or bird form that they admire. They can make sounds and mimic their movements, and write poetry or songs about the creature and how it relates to them. Using the mask's transformative power, the client can embody these qualities and strengths into their everyday life.

In exploring dreams and imagination, the mask can be transformed into a fantastical creature that represents the unconscious impulses, bringing them to the surface. The client can then make sounds and movements of this creature and create a dialogue to determine its wants and needs. The mask can also help to differentiate between a role that the client currently has versus what they would like to see happen. The mask can be designed to represent each of these values. Using the empty-chair technique, the client can explore each of these roles to help them decide on how to move forward with their choice.

The potential for exploration and transformation makes mask making a powerful clinical tool. It can provide an interpersonal dialogue between the client and the parts of their personality that are represented symbolically by the mask. Therapeutic mask making can also provide individuals with a tangible way to explore and articulate difficult thoughts, feelings, and emotions. Landy (1985) described the mask as a projective technique that provides objective distance between the masked part and the persona. Trepal-Wollenzier and Wester (2002) found that incorporating masks in a therapy session opens the space for the client to reflect on difficult issues while allowing them to be removed from the immediate situation behind the protection of the mask. Clients can then engage in a dialogue with the mask and enact a role play to work through and resolve any conflicts.

Consideration should be given to the client's cultural heritage, and research should be done on the historical context of these masks. Care should be taken to avoid appropriating other cultures when making masks and to instead focus on the client's heritage, which can also help to strengthen their sense of identity and help them find their authentic voice. Materials and media should be adapted to the client's developmental and cognitive abilities. Simplifying instructions and breaking the steps into smaller segments can help clients who need additional support. Masks can be simple or complex. They have the power to activate the imagination through play and can be used in a variety of ways. However, care should be taken to ensure that using masks and mask making is an appropriate intervention for specific clients because of their transformative power. For example, they might not be appropriate for clients who have lost touch with reality or are in an active psychotic break.

Conclusion

Historically, masks have been integral to the cultural practices of diverse populations and are used in a variety of rites and rituals. The mask possesses mystical-religious power and can be transformative. They can elicit an emotional response, shield the wearer's identity, and create the "other" persona. Masks and mask making have great potential as a therapeutic intervention because they can create objective distance and help clients to reflect on difficult issues while being protected by the mask. However, care should be taken to ensure that this is an appropriate intervention for specific clients and is contraindicated for clients who have lost touch with reality or who are experiencing a psychotic break.

References

Berlejeung, A., & Filitz, J. (Eds.). (2018). *The physicality of the other: Masks from the ancient near East and the Eastern Mediterranean.* Mohr Siebeck.

Dunn-Snow, P., & Joy-Smellie, S. (2000). Teaching art therapy techniques: Mask making, a case in point. *Journal of the American Art Therapy Association: Art Therapy, 17*(2), 125–131. https://doi.org/10.1080/07421656.2000.10129512

Edson, G. (2009). *Masks and masking: Faces of tradition and belief worldwide.* McFarland.

Elliott, B., & Conneller, C. (2020). Masks in context: Representation, emergence, motility and self. *World Archaeology, 52*(5), 655–666. https://doi.org/10.1080/00438243.2020.1996770

Foreman, J. (2000). *Maskwork.* The Lutterworth Press.

Harris, O. (2021). *Assembling past worlds: Materials, bodies and architecture in Neolithic Britain.* Routledge.

Hershman, D. (2014). *Face to face: The oldest masks in the world.* The Israel Museum.

Landy, R. J. (1985). The image of the mask: Implications for theatre and therapy. *Journal of Mental Imagery, 9*(4), 43–56. https://www.researchgate.net/publication/232419248

Landy, R. J. (1994). *Drama: Therapy concepts and practices.* Charles C. Thomas.

McNiff, S. (2004). *Art heals: How creativity cures the soul.* Shambhala.

Patterson, J., & Donahue, T. (2013). *Masks of the world.* Pearson.

Roy, D. (2000). Masks in pedagogical practice. *Journal for Learning Through the Arts, 12*(1), 1–12. http://escholarship.org/uc/item/83d8c84g

Roy, D. (2016). Masks as a method: Meyerhold to Mnouchkine. *Cogent Arts and Humanities, 3*(1), 1–11. https://doi.org/10.1080/23311983.2016.1236436

Sivin, C. (1986). *Mask making.* Davis.

Trepal-Wollenzier, H. C., & Wester, K. L. (2002). The use of masks in counseling. *Journal of Clinical Activities, Assignments and Handouts in Psychotherapy Practice, 2*(2), 123–130. https://doi.org/10.1300/J182v02n02_13

West, J. D., Watts, R. E., Trepal, H. C., Wester, K. W., & Lewis, T. F. (2001). Opening space for client reflection: A postmodern consideration. *The Family Journal, 9*(4), 431–437. https://doi.org/10.1177/1066480701094011

Chapter 2

I Contain Multitudes
Writing, Poetic Masks, and Parts of Self

Nancy S. Scherlong

Walt Whitman (1855) wrote, "I am large, I contain multitudes." Though many frequently associate the inception of masks with Greek theater (facially exaggerated images so audiences could better see the characters' features), the more accurate origin of masks is a "polyfunctional cultural phenomenon that was formed at the dawn of human civilization," inextricably linked to myth, ritual and transformation and imbued with a multitude of literal, societal/transactional, spiritual, and metaphorical meanings (Kirillova, 2022, p. 65). The field of anthropological knowledge of cultural masks is wide and deep and more than we can address here. It is worth stating that the creative arts, much like cultural masks, are indigenous practices, in existence before their colonization as professions. In literature, the use of mask and persona are almost interchangeable. In psychological terms, the Oxford Reference Dictionary defines *persona* as "the face that a person presents to the world, often derived from a sense of gender identity...stage of development...or occupation" (Hawkins, 2020). Across the lifespan, one may acquire a variety of different personas or, as Carl Gustav Jung would come to call them, "archetypes."

Jung (1959) believed that a persona could become pathological if one overidentified with it, was rigid in their adherence, or unable to adapt to changing circumstances. Both masks and metaphor, particularly in shamanic ritualized practice, hold the potential to transform one's inner and outer worlds, to loosen the bounds between self and other, energy and matter, and to create a liminal space for spiritual experiences to take place (Merrill, 2004). What or who do masks mask? What happens to parts of ourselves we wish for or idealize once the mask is removed? Are all masks chosen? How and when do they hide aspects that might bring judgement or violence or further oppression? What does the mask wearer see and how are they seen? What is missed or unseen? All of these are questions to be further explored through some of the poetry and writing we will encounter later.

DOI: 10.4324/9781003365648-4

Masks in Therapeutic Settings

Though nearly all the creative arts make some use of masks as an object or concept, they have been most prevalent in the therapeutic modalities of art, play, drama/psychodrama, and creative writing since the 1950s (Janzing, 1998). Drama therapist Robert Landy (1983, 1985) views the mask as mediator between the dual realities of daily life – the imaginal and the non-fiction – as well as a means through which to achieve aesthetic distance or separation between one's actual self and a character/role or part of self. Landy (1986) expounds on the power of masks to represent multiple sides of an issue, a means to explore identity in a group, to examine dreams, internalized imagery, or to express a social role.

Holistic Theories of Personality

There are quite a few multi-dimensional holistic models today of psycho-social functioning and identity formation. Many no longer feel bound by the old biologic theory of the mono-mind belief system, but instead now embrace the concept of subpersonalities; a term first coined in 1911 by Italian psychiatrist Alberto Assagioli (Rowan, 1990). Earlier, in the late 1800s, William James had spoken of the concept of internalized social selves based on a sense of group affiliation, a theory that left out important aspects of the multiplicity of belonging (Gaither, 2018). Of course, Freud had hinted at aspects of the psyche long before, but in a more fatalistic or restrictive manner than what has evolved over the past 40 years into a psycho-spiritual theoretical and practice model called Internal Family Systems theory (IFS).

IFS, founded by family systems therapist Dr. Richard Schwartz in the 1980s, posits the notion of an internalized system or multiplicity of selves or "parts," in which there are protectors (managers who are proactive and firefighters who are reactive) as well as vulnerable parts known as exiles. The aim of IFS, according to Schwartz (2021), is to achieve an integrated and relational understanding and self-connectedness, governed by the self (an innate center of calm and creativity and compassionate curiosity – among other traits). Surprisingly, not much has been written about the use of IFS principles within the fields of therapeutic writing or biblio-poetry therapy.

Metaphors and Mind

In the last 30 years, research on the power and significance of metaphor in the arts as well as in the world of advertising, linguistics, and human behavior has exploded. The Oxford Reference Dictionary defines *metaphor* as "a figure of speech in which a word or phrase is applied to an object or action to which it is not literally applicable" (Hawkins, 2020). The use of metaphors can be traced back (from Latin and French) to the 15th century with a root meaning of "to transfer." It is easy to see the unfolding of the mask as a metaphor or a means through which to transfer or project aspects of oneself or personality.

Metaphors, one of the most prominent literary poetic devices, are fundamental, pervasive, and naturally occurring ways in which we concretely and abstractly compare one thing to another, forging new meanings and connections (Lakoff & Johnson, 1980). Vicky Lai, a University of Arizona researcher, suggested that most people use a metaphor every 20 or so words. Using functional MRI's (magnetic resonance imaging technology), Lai et al. (2019) discovered that the understanding of metaphors may be centered in our physical experience; that an action metaphor like "grasp a concept" can also activate motor centers of the brain or encourage bi-hemispheric integration. Poetry and metaphor are both embodied and enacted, imbued with contextual and emotional significance, and rooted in experiential gestalts (Young, 2023). Young posits (akin to the theory of receptive biblio-poetry therapy) that poetic gestalts, much like metaphor, can be generalized to other experiences as a form of helping one to adapt to or negotiate challenging or unfamiliar life landscapes.

Theoretical Foundations and a Practice Model for Poetry Therapy (RES)

Bibliotherapy, or the use of stories, words, and literature to promote wellness or mental health, is an indigenous practice dating back to ancient times. The use of books to aid in adjustment and healing originates out of a library science tradition, though its most common therapeutic use today centers on interactive bibliotherapy, wherein materials are utilized for recognition, examination, juxtaposition, and application to the self through discussion and/or writing practices (Hynes & Hynes-Berry, 2012). It is worth noting that, unlike the tradition of literary criticism, bibliotherapy focuses on the emotional and cognitive impact of the work on the reader and the relevance of the material to their own past, present, or future lived experience rather than on the author's intent or meaning (Hynes & Hynes-Berry, 2012).

Poetry therapy, inclusive of bibliotherapy, is defined as the use of symbolic language in a therapeutic or educational context Mazza (2022). Modern poetry therapy, formally organized in the early nineteenth century, has roots in psychoanalytic, Jungian, Adlerian, cognitive-behavioral, gestalt, narrative, and constructivist theories and can therefore flexibly address the growing need for inclusive, non-binary structures (Mazza, 2022).

Mazza (1999) posits a tri-partite practice model for poetry therapy known as the RES:

- Receptive/prescriptive: Pre-existing poetry/literature is used to spark the interactive process.
- Expressive/creative: Generating writing occurs through a variety of prompts or questions.
- Symbolic/ceremonial: Metaphors, ritual, and storytelling enliven and enrich these connections.

Not every poetry therapy intervention will utilize all three of these phases, nor are they sequential or definite in nature. All the creative arts therapies contain these same thematic elements, which can be delivered along a continuum that is in close adherence to the unique developmental and clinical needs of the client or group. Selection of appropriate literature is perhaps one of the most complex aspects of biblio-poetry therapy. Some general guidelines include universality of theme and relatable emotion, striking or memorable imagery, clear and understandable language, compelling rhythm, and adequate complexity (Hynes & Hynes-Berry, 2012). In addition, the therapist considers the latent and manifest needs, explicit and implicit goals, as well as developmental and literacy level of the group or individual before embarking on a bibliotherapy intervention.

There are many guidelines in the literature for writing times – as long as 20 minutes in the classic expressive writing model (Pennebaker & Smyth, 2016) or as brief as five minutes in some journal therapy techniques (Adams, 1990). Often, less is more and it may be best to begin with tighter time frames for more emotionally laden material as well as to use an alarm system to cue when one has 30–60 seconds remaining to promote a sense of closure (Adams, 2013). Adding reflective practice to the writing experience (re-reading of one's work and response writing) can enrich insight, awareness, and self-understanding (Bolton & Delderfield, 2018).

Poetic Masks

Persona poetry (also known as mask poetry) is defined by the American Academy of Poetry as a style of dramatic monologue wherein the writer communicates through the voice of a fictional identity, character, or aspect of self or persona (Mabrouk, 2023). This poetic form assumes an audience but does not contain an interactive dialogue within the work itself. It is left to the reader to interpret the message, gauge its emotional passion, and impact (Mabrouk, 2023).

Perhaps the most frequently quoted poem about symbolic mask wearing is Paul Laurence Dunbar's (1895) "We Wear the Mask," in which the author refers to the masks of Blackness and oppression in America, that "We smile, but O great Christ, our cries... But let the world dream otherwise, / We wear the mask!" (p. 71). Persona poems can also serve as a type of dialogue between authors and across history, much like a character-based conversation. Writer and poet Maya Angelou, born 22 years after Dunbar's death, was so taken with this piece that she combined his original words with part of her own spoken word poem, entitled "The Mask," as viewed through the eyes of a Black woman she'd been observing on the bus and how her survival mask of laughter covered the depth of her pain and concealing their tears of submission (Hercules & Whack, 2017). Dunbar (1895) also had another poem entitled "Sympathy," from which the last line – "I know why the caged bird sings" (p. 102) – would later become the title for Angelou's autobiography.

Questions inspired in part by Schwartz's (2021) IFS model for learning more about protectors include:

- Reflecting upon your unique social identity and positionality, what masks have you, your family, or a part of yourself worn for protection or survival and how do they protect you? How old were you and what was happening when these masks came into being? What has been the function and impact of wearing the mask? With whom and when has it been safe enough to remove these masks?
- Who has inspired you from history? Borrow inspiration in the form of a line or image to begin your own persona poem.
- If your mask is one of privilege, how does being behind this mask (in whatever domain) impact how you see others, how they view you, and the opportunities that you encounter?
- Put on the mask of another who has vastly different lived experiences from yours, being sure to tune in with empathy, and write from their imagined perspective what a typical day might be like for them.

Another well-known poem on masks, simply entitled "Masks," is written by children's author Shel Silverstein (2011), in which two characters who both share a common trait (in this case, blue skin), go in search of someone like them and, because of the mask, never discover that they intersect. The meaning of this poem is not limited, of course, to just children and might lead to some interesting discussion or exploration through writing.

Additional questions for discussion or writing inspired in part by the IFS model for learning more about vulnerabilities or exiles (Schwartz, 2021):

- What is a trait or a part of yourself that you hide? Cultivate if you can, compassion from yourself toward this part. If you need to, tap into the positive regard that someone you know tends to have if it is hard to generate this from yourself.
- How does this part feel about you? What might if have to say to you right now?

- For how long and why has this part been hidden? How old were you when this part became hidden and what was happening that it felt it needed to do that?
- What would need to happen for you to feel safer, to reveal this part more, even just to yourself?

Other poems of note overtly mentioning masks include Muriel Rukeyser's (1967) "The Poem as Mask," a feminist consciousness work calling to dispel masks and mythologies put onto women which later inspired the anthology entitled *No More Masks!* (Howe & Bass, 1973). This anthology of nearly 100 female poets (spanning works written from 1919–1993) amplifies the voices of women writers writing about women's issues, their experience of a life self-divided, and their search for integration and wholeness in both their public and private worlds.

Also highly worth mentioning is the collection *A Face to Meet the Faces: An Anthology of Contemporary Persona Poetry* (Brown & de la Paz, 2012), a groundbreaking collection that takes a comprehensive look at persona poetry as a genre. The anthology's reach is wide, examining the writer's responses to historical and mythical events and figures, pop culture and celebrity, literary figures, and fairy tales as well as matters of social and political consciousness. Debora Kuan (2016) has an entire chapbook of poems exploring writing from the point-of-view of inanimate objects, food, and memories from her past. Yusef Komunyakaa's (2023) *Autobiography of My Alter Ego* and former poet laureate Billy Collins' (2014) TED Talk on "Two Poems on What Dogs Think (Probably)" are additional persona pieces worth investigating.

Writing Suggestion

Look around your environment. Notice what or who is nearby. Write your own persona poem from the imagined point of view of this object, person, pet. Take a moment to re-read your writing. What do you learn about yourself from this alternate perspective? How much of yourself is reflected in your descriptions? Reflect in writing, for a few sentences, about your observations.

Personification, List Making, and Plural Selves

Personification, the act of attributing human characteristics to inanimate or nonhuman objects or beings, is another form of metaphor (Lakoff & Johnson, 1980). The aesthetic distance provided by projecting parts of oneself onto the mask of character can free the speaker to be more imaginative, self-accepting, expressive, and vulnerable. *The Book of Qualities* (Gendler, 1988) is a wonderful collection of 78 such personifications or, as Adams

(1990) calls them, character sketches (and line drawings) that illuminate Depression's struggles, Anger's job as a knife sharpener, or Excitement's penchant for colorful socks.

The list poem is an old form that facilitates non-binary exploration, featuring the itemization of events, activities, or aspects of self (Padgett, 2000). Walt Whitman's (1855) *Song of Myself*, though not technically a persona poem, conveys through the description of both intensely personal and imagined universal experiences and its catalog-style of sweeping lists, a sense of identity that is layered and emphasizes the plural nature of the self. Carl Sandburg's (1970) poem includes an inventory of different animals and their traits that represent his multiplicitous identity.

Writing Suggestion

Make a list of some of your most-experienced emotional states or personality traits (or disowned ones). Write your own extended metaphor or personification of this feeling, remembering to include details such as appearance, attitude, dress, hopes, and fears. Re-reading what you wrote, what insights do you take away? How does this awareness impact your view of yourself now?

Conclusion

Rich opportunities exist for the exploration of the dynamic complexities of identity and the pluralistic self through examining metaphor and masks in poetry. Therapeutic gains of insight and self-awareness can be achieved through both reading and discussion, as well as through writing and reflection. There is far more to be discovered on the intersection of holistic psychology's theories of the multiplicity of mind and their examination through the lens of expressive writing and biblio-poetry therapy.

References

Adams, K. (1990). *Journal to the self: 22 paths to personal growth*. Warner Books.

Adams, K. (Ed.). (2013). *Expressive writing foundations of practice*. Rowman & Littlefield.

Bolton, G., & Delderfield, R. (2018). *Reflective practice: Writing and professional development*. SAGE Publications.

Brown, S. L., & De la Paz, O. (Eds.). (2012). *A face to meet the faces: An anthology of contemporary persona poetry*. The University of Akron Press.

Collins, B. (2014). *Two poems about what dogs think (probably)* [Video]. TED Talk. https://www.ted.com/talks/billy_collins_two_poems_about_what_dogs_think_probably

Dunbar, P. L. (1895). *The complete poems of Paul Laurence Dunbar*. Dodd, Mead, and Company.

Gaither, S. E. (2018). *The multiplicity of belonging: Pushing identity research beyond binary thinking*. Taylor & Francis.

Gendler, J. R. (1988). *The book of qualities*. Harper & Row.

Hawkins, J. M. (Ed.). (2020). *Metaphor*. Oxford Reference Dictionary. Retrieved March 31, 2023, from https://www.oxfordreference.com/display/10.1093/oi/authority.20110803100153175

Hercules, B., & Whack, R. C. (Dirs). (2017). *Maya Angelou: And still I rise* [Film]. PBS. https://www.pbs.org/video/american-masters-dr-maya-angelous-inspiration-and-poetry/

Howe, F., & Bass, E. (Eds.). (1973). *No more masks! An anthology of twentieth-century American women poets*. Anchor Books.

Hynes, A., & Hynes-Berry, M. (2012). *Biblio/poetry therapy, the interactive process: A handbook*. North Star Press.

Janzing, H. (1998). The use of the mask in psychotherapy. *Arts in Psychotherapy, 25*(3), 151–157. https://doi.org/10.1016/S0197-4556(98)00012-4

Jung, C. G. (1959). *Collected works of C. G. Jung: Archetypes and the collective unconscious* (R. F. C. Hull, Trans.). Princeton University Press.

Kirillova, N. B. (2022). Phenomenon of the mask as medium in history cultural. *Journal of the Belarusian State University, 4*(4), 63–71. https://doi.org/10.33581/2520-6338-2022-4-63-71

Komunyakaa, Y. (2023). *From autobiography of my alter ego*. https://poets.org/poem/autobiography-my-alter-ego

Kuan, D. (2016). *Lunch portraits*. Brooklyn Arts Press.

Lai, V., Howerton, O., & Desai, R. (2019). Concrete processing of action metaphors: Evidence from ERP. *Brain Research, 1714*, 202–209. https://doi.org/10.1016/j.brainres.2019.03.005

Lakoff, G., & Johnson, M. (1980). *Metaphors we live by*. University of Chicago Press.

Landy, R. J. (1983). The use of distancing in drama therapy. *The Arts in Psychotherapy, 10*(3), 175–185. https://doi.org/10.1016/0197-4556(83)90006-0

Landy, R. J. (1985). The image of the mask: Implications for theatre and therapy. *Journal of Mental Imagery, 9*(4), 43–56. https://psycnet.apa.org/record/1988-22929-001

Landy, R. J. (1986). *Drama therapy: Concepts and practices*. C.C. Thomas.

Mabrouk, N. (Ed.). (2023). *Persona: Explore the glossary of poetic terms*. https://poets.org/glossary/persona-poem

Mazza, N. (1999). *Poetry therapy: Interface of the arts and psychology*. CRC Press.

Mazza, N. (2022). *Poetry therapy: Theory and practice*. Routledge.

Merrill, M. (2004). Masks, metaphor and transformation: The communication of belief in ritual performance. *Journal of Ritual Studies, 18*(1), 16–33. http://www.jstor.org/stable/44368668

Padgett, R. (2000). *The teachers & writers handbook of poetic forms*. Teachers & Writers Collaborative.

Pennebaker, J. W., & Smyth, J. M. (2016). *Opening up by writing it down: How expressive writing improves health and eases emotional pain*. Guilford.

Rowan, J. (1990). *Subpersonalities: The people inside us*. Routledge.

Rukeyser, M. (1967). *The poem as mask: Orpheus*. Unicorn.

Sandburg, C. (1970). *The complete poems of Carl Sandburg*. Harcourt Brace.

Schwartz, R. C. (2021). *No bad parts*. Sounds True.

Silverstein, S. (2011). *Everything on it*. Penguin.

Whitman, W. (1855). *Leaves of grass*. American Renaissance.

Young, J. (2023). *Why poetry? Semiotic scaffolding & the poetic architecture of cognition*. Taylor & Francis.

Chapter 3

The Leelah Play

Avatar as Mask in Trauma-Informed Dramatherapy

Dov Blum-Yazdi

The Leelah Play (Blum-Yazdi, 2023) is a dramatherapy paradigm and a non-directive model. Avatar, a Sanskrit word, is related to the Jungian *persona*, which is designed to conceal the individual's true nature (Jung, 1953). The Leelah Avatar is an alter-ego which describes the client's role during the therapy sessions. The Leelah therapy is directed to the Avatar, not the player, meaning the Avatar is the one who gets the therapy. Some of the roots of trauma are intense physical or emotional reactions, avoiding thinking or talking about it, and dissociation strategies that allow clients to distance themselves from a situation that may otherwise be unbearable. Trauma symptoms continue when the real danger no longer exists, which can prolong or even prevent recovery. The Avatar works indirectly as a healing metaphor in trauma-informed dramatherapy. It helps clients move between situations smoothly and deal with trauma symptoms.

Trauma and Role-Play Post-Cult PTSD

Kai is in his late 20s; he joined Leelah's group therapy to help him deal with a voice disorder. From his early youth until age 25, Kai was part of a cooperative with a shared economy. In the cooperative, Kai worked as an educator in the periphery. They believe in social justice that focuses on land development for the benefit of all its citizens, on the foundations of freedom, justice, and peace. He voluntarily left the cooperative because of a ban on independent thinking.

Singer (1979) described the post-cult trauma syndrome (PCTS) as the intense emotional problems some members of cults and new religious movements experience upon disaffection and disaffiliation. PCTS is caused by deprogramming and is related to the consequences of leaving a cult. Some scholars in the field, including those critical of the anti-cult movement, acknowledge that abandoning a cult can be traumatic for some former members. Healy (2017) suggested that the prevalence of post-traumatic stress disorder (PTSD) is greater for former cult members than for any other

DOI: 10.4324/9781003365648-5

specific population. Additionally, "Former cult members experience a wide range of triggers, which reconnect the individuals with often-abhorrent cult experiences" (p. 62).

Early Trauma and Vocal Disorder

A few years after Kai left the cooperative, he was chronically hoarse. First, a wart was discovered on his vocal cords, which later turned out to be a polyp requiring surgical intervention. Eventually, he was diagnosed with a chronic disease called muscle tension dysphonia (MTD). MTD is frequently correlated with increased stress, anxiety, high demands, and feeling overwhelmed by commitments. In this sense, it is not unlike muscular tension throughout the rest of the body.

Baker (2003) reported an association between early trauma and vocal disorder. She found a relationship between psychogenic dysphonia (PDD) and earlier traumatic stress experienced some time before the onset of the dysphonia that seems to have been related to the recalling and telling of the narrative. PDD happens when a voice disorder has a psychic origin. It refers to the loss of voice when there is insufficient structural or neurological pathology to explain the nature and severity of the dysphonia and when the loss of voluntary control over the phonation appears to be related to psychological processes such as anxiety, depression, conversion reaction, or personality disorder (Rosen et al., 2020). Van der Kolk (2014) felt that you can use role-play and access your inner sensations to find your voice, which is the opposite of dissociation, of being out of the body and disappearing. According to him, traumatized people are afraid to meet deep feelings. They are terrified to meet those feelings because it brings them back to the trauma. Therefore, "theater is about embodying emotions, giving voice to them, becoming rhythmically engaged, taking on and embodying different roles" (p. 335).

Trauma-Informed Role-Play Method

At some point, a protest by former members and parents of the cooperative compared it to Scientology and depicted their lifestyle as cult-like while accusing them of employing social pressure and manipulation to keep their members. For example, refusing academic studies because academia is capitalist, restricting military service, and prohibiting travel abroad. These restrictions were intended to make sure that members stick to the cooperative framework, with their people and ideas, and not to be tempted by the outside world.

Based on widely divergent fields of psychotherapy, social advocacy, and basic science, psychological abuse, neglect, and trauma continue to be at the center of drama therapists' attention. Dramatherapy's contribution to this pervasive effort to address psychological trauma in social policy, advocacy, treatment, and education is significant. Dramatherapy has primarily been applied towards personal development in educational settings and towards ameliorating psychiatric symptoms among hospitalized patients. Dramatherapy has been engaged in treating both individual and collective trauma (Johnson & Sajnani, 2014).

According to the American Psychological Association, one of the leading PTSD symptoms is dissociation (VandenBos, 2007). Dissociation in response to actual traumatic events can be triggered, even long afterward, by events that may or may not be threatening. Role-based methods allow for the exploration of trauma roles to build a reflective understanding of rigid characterizations and reintegrate that which has been dissociated (Haen & Weber, 2009). "Exploring dissociation through a dramatic lens necessarily begins with an exploration of role" (Hodermarska et al., 2014, p. 182).

Jones (2015) explores how role-play features in dramatherapy's engagement with clients who have experienced trauma. He argues that role-playing and playfulness are key parts of the ways in which dramatherapy can offer help. Armstrong et al. (2019), indicated that role-play had the greatest positive impact for those with neurological trauma or degeneration, older adults, social justice, and trauma. Additionally, they present an analysis that points out impairment decreasing in an experimental group, indicating that engagement in a role-play story elicits the most significant positive impact.

Landy (1993) argues that each person is a composite of aesthetic roles, somatic, cognitive, affective, social/cultural, and spiritual, constituting a role system. Throughout this perspective, he presents a role taxonomy, "a theatrical archetype system" consisting in its original form of 84 role types (p. 163). Drama therapy approaches based on role theory potentially mitigate the deadness of trauma by offering up discoveries of "internal and relational strength" held and expressed within stories and roles (Landy, 2010, p. 10).

Leelah's Avatar

I describe the Leelah Play as a dramaturgic therapeutic method that uses play for therapy, combining theories of drama with classical psychoanalytic concepts. The Leelah Play consists of two parts: the Leelah Play Paradigm – a theory that redefines terms such as power relationship, freedom, and identity of the playing person in therapy. Leelah Play for Itself – an application of the Leelah Play Paradigm based on undirected role-play within the frame of a long-term narrative. This model suggests a therapeutic process of non-intervention, an autonomous and self-healing work led by the players themselves, where the play stands for itself, and the therapist's position is phenomenological (Blum-Yazdi, 2017). Leelah addresses the role of the impact of trauma in dramatherapy through long-term and profound role-play. Hence, Leelah's unique contribution is using Avatar as therapy for traumatic situations. The sessions can be individual or group, while the therapist uses an Avatar herself. My Avatar name in this case study was Raul.

The therapist creates the general initial story and provides a general framework and rules. The rest of the plot is devised interactively by the characters that develop during the play. Few scenes are happening simultaneously and creating a playful space in an imaginary town, in this case named Gimignano, which is an open space and is unpredictable since each character's actions depend on random actions and the autonomous decisions of the player.

After each session, Leelah's players report in their diaries and verbally share the experiences of their Avatars. This is Kai's Avatar diary's first report:

"Saladin is a 32-year-old who was born in the town of Barga and, until recently, lived with his two elderly parents. He had studied physics but dropped out and chose to become a junior sultan so that he could continue his parents' heritage. 18 months ago, he finished his junior sultan training and was certified. Recently, his parents stationed him in Gimignano. This meant that he still had to move far away from them. Unfortunately, since moving, he does not see them very often, but is able to stay in touch."

Step One – Developmental Sequences

This is Kai's Avatar diary's second report:

> Saladin has been able to establish relationships with the townspeople and has joined a weekly archery class. When the townspeople listen to him and everything is in order, he is connected to townsfolks, tolerant, highly motivated in his duty and enjoys life. When the townspeople do not listen to him, he sinks into despair and grows withdrawn, detached, and intolerant.

The core clinical aspect of Leelah is working with the developmental sequences (DS) of the Avatar. The Leelah Play draws on the triple-spiral triskelion, an ancient Celtic symbol, as a form of the psyche of the Avatar. Each of these three spirals is a staircase spiral. Each stair represents a linear component and the spiral structure in which they are embedded represents the cyclic component. In Leelah, therapy works by establishing three DS for each of the three spirals. The spectrum is structured as a linear oxymoron, which contains contradictions and paradoxes. In this structure, movement is subjected to the Aristotelian law which states that motion occurs between relevant opposites (Barnes & Aristotle, 2014). When an Avatar is preoccupied with a certain theme, the opposing theme is also necessarily relevant to them, even if it is not tangibly manifest at first. In Saladin's case, following his report, I chose detached/connected.

Step Two – Four Types of Movement

The three sequences remain the same throughout the therapy. They accompany the Avatar during every session and constitute its key characteristic. The only person consciously aware of them and monitoring them is the therapist. Within each oxymoron, the paradigm defines four types of movement that portray the dialogue between its two poles: (a) blocked, (b) sudden, (c) hesitant, and (d) harmonic (Figure 3.1).

At the end of each session, the therapist uses these icons to mark the relevant type of movement on the individual developmental sequences tracker (DST), which is meant for the therapist alone. The therapist's goal is to enable each Avatar to become acquainted with all four movement types. In Saladin's DST, I noted detached/connected as the first sequence and marked "blocked" for movement since his feeling was mainly detached and withdrawn.

All four movements are equally important for healing trauma and are not in any hierarchical relationship with one another. The sequences are designed to disrupt any oppressive dynamic by which the therapist favors the integrative pole over the dissociative one and directs the player towards a particular point on the spectrum. The paradigm wishes to move beyond the linear-hierarchical view and replace it with a circular/spiral one (Blum-Yazdi, 2013). This encounter between opposite poles creates a spinning structure, which heals the trauma.

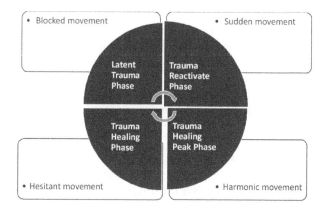

Figure 3.1 Trauma phase.

Leelah defines the Latent Trauma Phase as a state in which a client's status movement is blocked. The Trauma Reactivate Phase happens when the triggers are pushed and the movement changes into sudden movement. The Trauma Healing Phase starts when the client discovers the hesitant movement by themselves, not by the therapist leading. The goal is to enable the client to go through dissociation and integration situations and to allow them both. The Trauma Healing Peak Phase happens when the movement is harmonic, and both poles meet. The order between the phases is not necessarily chronological. In the next section, I will demonstrate those phases.

Step Three – Trauma Care Through Avatar

After some sessions playing the Leelah, Kai's trauma events came up; at this stage, my out-role therapy connection with Kai, as needed, became individual as well. During the process after play, he first began to speak about his voice disorder as a technical problem. I asked him if he remembered a similar situation of speaking difficulty, and he remembered memories from his period in the cooperative. It was the first time the connection between Kai's voice disorder and the cooperative life was made.

Processing Kai's Perspective. Meanwhile, in Gimignano, the authorities decided on town renovation. Let us read Kai's Avatar's report:

> Due to town renewal, the townspeople started talking about the place they are planning to move to, Saladin mustered up his courage and stated that he suggested that they should all prepare for a rebellion to stay. This may be the first time that Saladin voiced such a clear-cut opinion in the town forum.

As the last section showed, the previous Saladin movement was blocked in the detached pole, meaning the trauma was in the Latent Phase. One can notice the spontaneous reconciliation between Saladin and the townsfolk, representing the cooperative members, and the sudden shift towards the connected pole. As Kai reported, it was "the first time"; therefore, I marked "sudden" for movement in the DST. This scene demonstrates the Trauma Reactivation Phase and parallels Kai's recalling of the cooperative period, as Kai stated:

> There was no independent thinking but dictates of the way of thinking to the point of brainwashing. For example, we read and quoted by heart collections of texts, Martin Buber's group ideas. We talked tirelessly about group life, ideals, society, and against exploiting workers. I tried to bring my unique ideas to the cooperative, but my voice was never heard.

The cooperative was demanding and stressful while canceling the self to the point of helplessness. Kai's vocal disorder resulted from prolonged exposure to self-sacrificing relationships, self-abnegation, and damaged his ability to form trusting relationships.

Re-Processing Kai's Perspective. In Kai's Avatar report, Saladin thinks about retiring from his role as junior Sultan:

> It suddenly occurred to Saladin...how great it would be...to leave his exhausting role as junior sultan and maybe go back to his study of physics, which he had abandoned. This thought filled him with a comforting sense of nostalgia as well as sadness over all the things he is about to leave...once again, the delicious memory of the cookies his father would make came to Saladin's mouth...Raul's curiosity [also] felt pleasant, because he felt his intentions were good....When they sat around the bonfire, Saladin was once again overwhelmed by a strong feeling of warmth....[A]ll the townspeople ate and enjoyed themselves very much....Knowing that he could take care of himself empowered and comforted him.

The Trauma Healing Phase begins with hesitant movement, which is expressed in the comforting, moderate, and grounded feeling in this scene. Therefore, this time I marked "hesitant" in the DST. However, the process is not linear. Saladin moved back and forth along the fourth phase and dealt with issues from different steps, which made his process both profound and authentic. Kai, post factum, re-realized that he never liked being an educator or a leader as he was asked to. In Kai's words:

"I realized the world's fate does not rest on my shoulders; I don't have to fight everyone else's wars, and the world probably won't collapse because of my herd. If, in the past, I trained everyone to be a leader, I discovered that not everyone was meant for it; the discovery was shocking."

I wish to stress that, as a therapist, I had no preference for the positive pole. My Avatar Raul's presence was supportive, protective, and non-judgmental towards any movement. Those conditions made it possible for Saladin to become acquainted with additional forms of movement and the Avatar was able to undergo a process of self-regulation and spontaneous healing. The Trauma Healing Phase started when Saladin discovered the hesitant movement by himself, not by my leading.

Re-Processing Kai's Farewell. Back to the Gimignano town plot, Kai's Avatar following report describes Saladin's farewell ceremony:

> As a tribute to his town departure, Saladin took the bread, which he baked for the townspeople, out of the oven...and invited his friend to join him in giving it to everyone. They met the neighbors, who had some bread

with jam. Saladin offered some bread to Raul…and then to the peddler and the elder as well. All town residents stood in a circle, conversing. Saladin felt a deep sense of warmth, feeling that they were like a family.

We can see Saladin decided to leave the town and began his preparations for concluding his stay there. In the last excerpt, one can note Saladin's developmental movement, which became possible through the support he received and the acceptance of his full range of qualities. He could detach from the townsfolk and simultaneously connect to a new place. Therefore, this time I marked "harmonic" on the DST.

In our private conversation, Kai said:

> We worked from morning to evening for the sake of fulfilling an ideal. It was forbidden to say it was difficult. As a result, some members had a nervous breakdown and suddenly retired without explanation or saying goodbye. After many years of sharing my life with the members, I decided to leave. When I announced my retirement, I got a message that I had chosen darkness, a life of corruption, and money pursuit. A parting process was not allowed; my friends immediately turned their back on me and treated me as a traitor.

Notice that the Trauma Healing Peak Phase happens when the movement is harmonic and both poles meet. When Saladin spontaneously went through dissociation-integration (detached-connected), he could disconnect (a dissociation quality) his location in Gimignano, using an integration quality, to find his best relocation. Receiving the townsfolk's support during his leaving was a corrective experience, replacing the abandonment of his cooperative friends, and healing his cooperative traumatic wound.

Conclusion

In conclusion, one should be "mindful of the potential for flooding or dissociation, resulting in the risk of re-traumatizing in the process" (Chadwick, 2021, p. 119). However, desensitizing Kai to the trauma issues enables him to stabilize, self-regulate, and process trauma without activating the symptoms (Barbato, 1945). Moreover, desensitization no longer serves as a focus of anxiety since Kai's procedure was one of catharsis. The establishment of a safe environment for play, without an audience, external goals, or interpretation, creates a secure social laboratory for PTSD. This environment allows players to bring up important clinical material that was forgotten in the case of dissociation. The therapist's presence is not the dominant one and is instead focused on maintaining and holding the healing of the traumatic space.

I would like to thank Gidi Zehavi for the intellectual dyad forum and the rich discussions on drama therapy.

Reference

Armstrong, C. R., Frydman, J. S., & Rowe, C. (2019). A Snapshot of empirical drama therapy research: Conducting a general review of the literature. *GMS Journal of Arts Therapies*, *1*, 1–16. https://www.egms.de/static/en/journals/jat/2019-1/jat000002.shtml

Baker, J. (2003). Psychogenic voice disorders and traumatic stress experience: A discussion paper with two case reports. *Journal of Voice*, *17*(3), 308–318. https://doi.org/10.1067/S0892-1997(03)00015-8

Barbato, L. (1945). Drama therapy. *Sociometry*, *8*(3/4), 158–160. https://doi.org/10.2307/2785039

Barnes, J., & Aristotle (2014). *The complete works of Aristotle: The revised Oxford translation* (J. L. Ackrill, Trans.). Princeton University Press.

Blum-Yazdi, D. (2013). Language, Kwan, world. *Journal of East-West Psychology*, *3*(39), 1-14.https://www.academia.edu/44315071/Language_Koan_World

Blum-Yazdi, D. (2017). *Drama therapy Leelah – A non-directive model* [Video]. YouTube. https://www.youtube.com/watch?v=pY26_T4Zqts

Blum-Yazdi, D. (2023). Leelah play. In M. Hills de Zarate, S. Pitruzzella & U. Herrmann (Eds.), *Arts therapies and the mental health of children and young people: Contemporary research, theory and practice*. Routledge.

Chadwick, E. M. (2021). Beauty and the beast: Trauma-informed dramatherapy with a male patient in a forensic setting. In S. Hastilow & M. Liebmann (Eds.), *Arts therapies and sexual offending* (pp. 115–134). Jessica Kingsley Publishers.

Haen, C., & Weber, A. M. (2009). Beyond retribution: Working through revenge fantasies with traumatized young people. *The Arts in Psychotherapy*, *36*(2), 84–93. https://doi.org/10.1016/j.aip.2009.01.005

Healy, D. P. (2017). The unique characteristics of post cult post-traumatic stress disorder and suggested therapeutic approaches. *International Journal of Cultic Studies*, *8*, 60–70. https://psycnet.apa.org/record/2017-24020-005

Hodermarska, M., Haen, C., & McLellan, L. (2014). Exquisite corpse: On dissociation and intersubjectivity–implications for trauma-informed drama therapy. In N. Sajnani & D. R. Johnson (Eds.), *Trauma-informed drama therapy: Transforming clinics, classrooms, and communities* (pp. 179–205). Charles C. Thomas.

Johnson, D. R., & Sajnani, N. (2014). The role of drama therapy in trauma treatment. In N. Sajnani & D. R. Johnson (Eds.), *Trauma-informed drama therapy* (pp. 5–23). Charles C. Thomas Publisher.

Jones, P. (2015). Trauma and dramatherapy: Dreams, play and the social construction of culture. *South African Theatre Journal*, *28*(1), 4–16. https://doi.org/10.1080/10137548.2015.1011897

Jung, C. G. (1953). *Collected works of C. G. Jung, Volume 7: Two essays on analytical psychology* (G. Adler & R. F. C. Hull, Trans.). Princeton University Press.

Landy, R. J. (1993). The child, the dreamer, the artist and the fool: In search of understanding the meaning of expressive therapy. *The Arts in Psychotherapy*, *20*(5), 359–370. https://doi.org/10.1016/0197-4556(93)90043-2

Landy, R. J. (2010). Drama as a means of preventing post-traumatic stress following trauma within a community. *Journal of Applied Arts and Health*, *1*(1), 7–18. https://doi.org/10.1386/jaah.1.1.7/1

Rosen, D. C., Shmidheiser, M. H., Sataloff, J. B., Hoffmeister, J., & Sataloff, R. T. (2020). Psychogenic dysphonia. In D. C. Rosen, J. B. Sataloff, & R. T. Sataloff (Eds.), *Psychology of voice disorders* (pp. 187–207). Plural Publishing.
Singer, M. T. (1979, January). Coming out of the cults. *Psychology Today*, 72–81. https://articles1.icsahome.com/articles/coming-out-of-cults-singer
Van der Kolk, B. (2014). *The body keeps the score: Brain, mind, and body in the healing of trauma*. Viking.
VandenBos, G. R. (Ed.). (2007). *APA dictionary of psychology*. American Psychological Association.

Chapter 4

A Transformative Journey of Masks in Drama Therapy

Reversing the Sequence in Lecoq's Physical Theater Pedagogy

Shiu Hei Larry Ng

Jacques Lecoq (1921–1999) used different types of masks in his actor-creator pedagogy for physical theater. On the one hand, drama therapy works through dramatically structured and theatrically mediated experiential processes of embodied imagination and/or imaginative embodiment for people's transformation. On the other hand, in Lecoq's pedagogy, mime as *mimodynamics* is embodiment and embodied cognition/experience with the mask as an incomplete, dynamic structure, with masking as the interface/mediation between embodiment and imagination. From my practical experience in both physical theater and drama therapy working with youth and adults, I reversed Lecoq's pedagogical sequence to help clients make layer-by-layer inner improvement and transformation systematically, with the help of different types of masks one after another. This is different from how masks are usually used in drama therapy and hence can enrich the application of masks in this therapeutic practice. Clinically, masks can provide strong containment and function as catalysts of amplification and condensation of experience for different kinds of therapeutic activation and transformation, so they make different healing processes happen with higher speed and higher safety. Using ready-made masks does not exclude nor ignore the fact that they can trigger psychological associations based on personal life experiences and memories, mediated by one's own and social-cultural background, as well as the fact that they have archetypal and symbolic-ritualistic potentials that can channel huge transpersonal power.

Mask as a Portable Dynamic Structure to be Completed by the Body

A mask is usually used as a projective tool, like puppets, dolls, and symbolic objects, while its image of a face gives a stronger effect in relation to themes like identity and emotion. The common way to use masks in drama therapy is usually to guide clients to make their own mask as a visual art piece, often by putting a collage of colored papers, drawings, paintings, and other

DOI: 10.4324/9781003365648-6

accessories on a white mask, plate, or paper bag, or sometimes by sculpting a face in clay. Imagination, association, and psychological projection naturally happen during the creative process of mask making. After the mask is made, there is a second layer of experience when clients put on their masks and imagine themselves becoming the mask character and embodying this character through movement and dance, or even making the mask play as a ritual. Using ready-made masks is much rarer comparatively speaking because the first layer of experience and projection during the mask making process is absent/skipped, and the personal connection to the mask is much weaker.

However, inspired by Amleto Sartori, masks used in Lecoq's pedagogy must be structurally sculpted and suggest certain dynamics to be effective on stage by pushing the space in certain ways and projecting its dynamic structure to the space. Such masks are an incomplete structure to be animated by the player's body, so the wearer also needs to push the space with their gestures and movements in specific ways. Thus, an effective mask influences its wearer primarily in a physical way that corresponds to its shape and, more precisely, to the inherent dynamics suggested by the shape on an embodiment level (Estévez, 2015). This is essentially the difference between a ready-made sculptural mask (by a trained, skillful mask maker) and the visual mask made by untrained clients (usually with limited skills). The latter is a visual object behind which the wearer moves according to their memory, impression, or association of the mask's visual appearance as it is seen from the outside. In the former, the wearer is motivated and guided by the sculptural mask as it is seen from the outside and its dynamic structure from within, not just visually but also spatially and kinesthetically.

Reversing Lecoq's Sequence for Improvisation Exploration

Lecoq's pedagogy uses different types of masks in a particular progressive sequence for improvisational exploration, which starts with the neutral mask, and then larval masks, expressive masks, commedia dell'arte half-masks, and finally red noses (Lecoq, 2000, 2006; Wright, 2002). Lecoq's pedagogical reason for this sequence design was to guide students from a state of balance to different types of off-balance in space and decrease the size of the face area covered by the mask step by step. However, from my experiences with clients, I found that following Lecoq's pedagogical sequence was too hard and abstract for clients to start with the neutral mask. In comparison, starting with the commedia dell'arte half-masks is the most convenient and friendly entrance because they are fun, much easier to use and the least scary for people without any experience of wearing/playing with a mask.

In existing practices, the major principles/mechanisms of using masks therapeutically can be summarized as follows (see Table 4.1):

Table 4.1 Principle or mechanism for the use of masks in drama therapy

Principle/Mechanism	Origins/References
projection	psychoanalysis, depth psychology
distancing/playing of distance (interpersonal and intrapsychic)	sociology (symbolic interactionism), social psychology
ritual transformational trance	spiritual practices/traditions, anthropology

According to Landy (1985) and Napier (1986), the principles/mechanism of using masks in drama therapy include empowerment, flexibility (e.g., shifting among roles and expansion of role repertoire, etc.), and the capacity/wisdom to contain/stay with paradoxes (e.g., living with tensions of opposites or ambiguity in-between, or individuating the universal, etc.). Through this process, masks are used as instruments of "metamorphosis/transformer" and "channel/mediator" (Rolfe, 1977; Hutchison, 2011).

However, compared with this summary, Lecoq's unique dynamic approach to masks does not apply any of the above mechanisms. Therefore, his pedagogy can be a reference for a new approach to how masks can be used in drama therapy. It can theoretically illustrate and practically demonstrate:

1. How drama/theater is grounded in our sensorimotor being and emerges from playful embodiment.
2. How metaphor emerges from movement and can be used intentionally and systematically as a way of creating metaphorical connections and communicating the natural, social, psychological, and even the transpersonal (especially when Greek Tragedy and Buffon are explored in the second year of Lecoq's pedagogy).

Lecoq's pedagogy is also significant to drama therapy in that it does not rely on any psychological, sociological, or spiritual theories/explanations/traditions to understand theater and mask, as it is basically phenomenological and practical. Therefore, it can merge with existing drama therapy models based on particular theories.

Stage One: Commedia Dell'Arte Half-Masks

Commedia dell'arte half-masks are easier and less scary to start with, not only because they are dynamically bold and look fun/comic, but also because they cover only half of the face (Figure 4.1). It is less difficult for clients to breathe under half-masks as the mouth is uncovered, and hence they also encourage/suggest the use of voice besides movement. They demonstrate

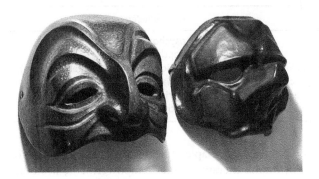

Figure 4.1 Commedia dell'arte half-masks.

Photographed by Shiu Hei Larry Ng.

clearly the amplification effect of the mask in general, and the important fact that a mask can only be brought alive by the player (because without a player, the mask is not even a complete face), so the player is always the one who decides to engage or not.

For additional safety, clients are invited to choose a mask that they want to explore and then go in pairs with another client, taking turns to put their chosen mask on their partner's face first, and then guide/teach the masked partner how to move using particular gestures and rhythm before the partner can get a sense of the dynamics and accordingly, they can move independently. Only after this process, can clients then play with the mask individually, in pairs or in trios in some commedia dell'arte scenarios, which are kept short/brief with a high turnover rate. The exaggerated comic scenes usually induce a lot of laughter, playfulness, and energy.

Clinically, these half-masks can help clients to get into big body gestures and physically reconnect with their primitive life-force/vitality and desire, under the containment of playfulness. These energies are channeled by the stock characters into a flow of resilient, flexible, and witty responsiveness for both survival and enjoyment/desire-fulfillment. It opens a horizon beyond good and evil, under which life itself or even fate is embraced with an energetic "yes," and thus it can also increase clients' tolerance to the "shadow" materials in the Jungian sense and help them to play with/ around oppression or power asymmetry. All these are important resources/ strengths crucial for the upcoming deeper work for therapy, and clients can recollect/redevelop them via impersonal play full of fun and energy.

Stage Two: Expressive Masks

Expressive masks are full masks covering the whole face, with a sculptural-dynamic feature that can make us imagine a face with more than one emotional expression, with conflicting emotions, or a state in the middle of two or more expressions. Therefore, it also looks like they get stuck in between emotions, or that they try to hide/suppress their expressions but cannot help leaking out some. Consequently, "suppressive mask" would be an even more suitable name. The body with expressive mask reacts to situations physically with reservation and/or subtlety. Dynamically opposite to commedia dell'arte half-masks, expressive masks need only very small, subtle movement to bring them alive, and they can sustain a longer pause that is vibrant. The traces/features of the "face" can also be understood as a distortion because of both external and internal forces that are overwhelming but beyond one's own will. These characteristics make expressive masks perfect for clients to get in touch obliquely with personal wounds and emotional/sentimental sufferings, under a poetic containment.

Short existential scenes of universal sentimental themes of humanity, like separation/loss, conflicts in intimacy, individual-collective struggle, etc., can be played out with masks in a condensed manner to highlight certain moments or under an additional protection by a dramaturgy of selecting scenes that are just a bit "off" from the most intense drama, as in Chekhov's plays. They call for and contain feelings/sentiments around loss and/or lack, including direct feelings/sentiments, sadness and anger, and other more indirect, complicated feelings like regret, shame, and resentment. As the core of such usually suppressed complex of feelings/sentiments is loss/lack, the double containment of masks plus poetic dramaturgy allows an oblique mourning process to occur, which is key to free clients from the curse-like/ghost-like emotional/sentimental entanglement and for any further transformation to happen (Bowlby, 1980; George et al., 2023; Kavaler-Adler, 2004).

After/during later parts of this "poetic mourning" process, ritual elements are added. Clients are invited to create a ritual, or a ritual scene/action, either *with* the mask on or *for/to* the mask when the mask is not worn but used like a special object or part of an installation. Through such a ritual, clients can bring the mourning to a closure and get ready for a new beginning. Clients are invited to tour around a "world" with this type of mask, either wearing the mask with a larger distance between the mask and them or hold the mask like the head of a puppet, to prevent overidentification for safety and imagine a transpersonal character represented by this mask, be it a god, fairy, or supernatural being. Such play opens a transpersonal/cosmic horizon to contain and further digest personal-existential materials in the poetic play and the ritualistic play. Thus, in this stage, there is a three-fold movement from the personal/existential-poetic via the ritualistic to the transpersonal.

Stage Three: Larval Masks

Larval masks have large and bold shapes with lots of roundedness and are a transitional type/state between expressive masks and neutral masks because they have no clear "face," but their shapes keep making us imagine faces that are out of balance/calmness (Figure 4.2). They also have child-like/cartoon-like features, and they can also be seen as a face/personality in their formation and hence a transitional, immature state with certain directionality, full of potentials. They invite players to use simple but clear movements to bring them alive. It is a mask of pure play, and it echoes an innocent state of being before any trauma/impact of downfall. In such a state, people have a pure curiosity to simply explore the world around them and learn.

According to Winnicott (1991), the first level of play with these masks is pure play with curiosity, simplicity, and direct reactions, in which clients can reconnect to their core vitality of growth and creativity. Such play has an effect like a kind of developmental repair for clients. The second level with these masks is more "psychodramatic." In turns, one client with a larval mask on is placed on stage to play a child character, and other participants without masks enter the stage one after another to play different roles interacting with this child. Very often, in such improvisation, these other

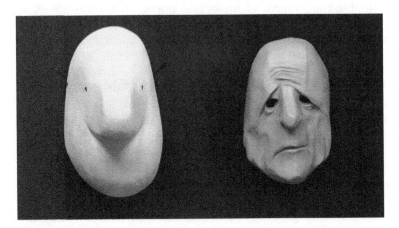

Figure 4.2 Larval and expressive masks.
Photographed by Shiu Hei Larry Ng.

characters happen to be adult roles, and, surprisingly, such adult roles are usually cruel or unfriendly ones. Therefore, plays about children in adversities or even traumatized children usually appear.

These scenes have impacts on both the players with and without masks, and equally on the participants who are audiences. In small groups, each client has a chance to invite and instruct other group members to act as the "ideal parents" for that child character represented by the larval mask they have chosen, and they later put on the mask to become the child character, interacting with the ideal parents to receive/experience/enjoy the care they need. After that, to get closer to the complexity of reality for their maturation process, "good-enough parents" instead of "ideal parents" are explored in similar ways. Therefore, this stage is about retrieving the innermost innocence, nurturing this core for growth, and supporting clients to grow (once again) from this core, allowing the healing/transformative process to be embodied through the containment and articulation of mask plays (Kalsched, 2013).

Stage Four: Neutral Masks

The neutral mask is different from a dead white mask with no expression or a Buddha's calm face with a certain degree of detachment; instead, it is a mask of readiness and openness, moving towards the whole space/world and being one with everything, although the word "neutral" often misleads people to think about being "disinterested" or "detached" (see Figure 4.3).

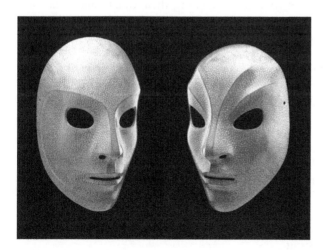

Figure 4.3 Male and female neutral masks.
Photograph by the Sartori family.

Specially designed by Sartori, the neutral mask is the first mask to be explored in Lecoq's pedagogical sequence for training actor-creators, preparing them to be open and ready enough to receive inspiration from the moving world and enter different explorations. In therapy, neutral masks are used for the second-to-last stage to help clients integrate the discoveries and therapeutic experiences in previous stages, helping them reach a state of openness and readiness to fully re-enter the outer world from the inner journey after (a) the primitive life-force is reactivated and rechanneled (via commedia dell'arte half-masks), (b) the stuck sentiments are released and transformed (via expressive masks), and (c) the innocent core of vitality and creativity for growth is reawakened and allowed to redevelop (via larval masks).

In short, it is a mask for both inner integration/coordination and outer engagement in its fullness, and for a dynamic balancing (or, say, harmony) between the inner and outer experiential processes. It is crucial therapeutically for clients to keep the newly tuned inner state while gradually stepping into the outer world for exploration, adventure, and creation again.

Stage Five: Red Nose

The red nose of clown, which is the smallest mask in the world, has the power to highlight the uniqueness of a person's face and also the whole body. It is the last stage for both Lecoq's physical theater pedagogy and for this therapy journey in the author's practices. Theatrically, it is used to help actor-creators in training discover their uniqueness, which is their most important creative resource. Therapeutically, it is used to help clients to explore their unique ways of individuating their vitality and creativity, flowing from their innermost core of growth, together with their life-forces and existential feelings, in the context of reality. Both theatrically and therapeutically, embracing fully and creatively one's uniqueness and whole self, including the vulnerable parts and the usually unaccepted parts, is a necessary step to conclude and consolidate growth. The red nose is a mask for such an important state to complete the transformational process.

Conclusion

Different layers of self-exploration correspond to different types of masks. This layer-by-layer process of self-exploration/transformation can also be seen as a sequence of:

1. Resourcing/Grounding
2. Processing/Digesting
3. Refreshing/Rebirth

4. Integrating/Harmonizing
5. Individuating

Such mask-driven/led embodiment and exploration can touch upon different levels/layers of self, existence, humanity, and psyche, stage by stage. This is made possible by using different types of masks available in Lecoq's physical theater pedagogy, but in almost a reversed order. This is due to therapeutic considerations for the needs and conditions of clients, which are very different from theater students. This approach is not based on psychological projection and association, but on dynamic embodiment that grounds imagination, emotions, and other psychological processes. In other words, it is a kind of psyche transformation/psychological change that is physically founded. It expands the possibility of the use of masks in drama therapy.

References

Bowlby, J. (1980). *Attachment and loss: Loss, sadness and depression* (Vol. 3). Basic Books.

Estévez, C. (2015). Mask performance for a contemporary Commedia dell'arte. In J. Chaffe & O. Crick (Eds.), *The Routledge companion to commedia dell'arte* (pp. 130–138). Routledge.

George, C., Aikins, J. W., & Lehmann, M. (2023). *Working with attachment trauma: Clinical application of the adult attachment projective picture system.* Taylor & Francis.

Hutchison, Y. (2011). Mask today: Mediators of a complex reality. *South African Theatre Journal, 8*(1), 45–62. https://doi.org/10.1080/10137548.1994.9688109

Kalsched, D. (2013). *Trauma and the soul: A psycho-spiritual approach to human development and its interruption.* Routledge.

Kavaler-Adler, S. (2004). *Mourning, spirituality and psychic change: A new object relations view of psychoanalysis.* Routledge.

Landy, R. J. (1985). *Essays in drama therapy: The double life.* Jessica Kingsley.

Lecoq, J. (2000). *The moving body.* Bloomsbury Methuen Drama.

Lecoq, J. (2006). *Theatre of movement and gesture.* Routledge.

Napier, A. D. (1986). *Masks, transformation, and paradox.* University of California Press.

Rolfe, B. (1977). *Behind the mask.* Charlemagne Press.

Winnicott, D. W. (1991). *Playing and reality.* Psychology Press.

Wright, J. (2002). The masks of Jacques Lecoq. In F. Chamberlain & R. Yarro (Eds.), *Jacques Lecoq and the British theatre* (pp. 71–84). Routledge.

Chapter 5

Integrating Voice Movement Therapy and Mask Work and Why it Works

Gina Holloway Mulder

Voice movement therapy (VMT) is an expressive arts therapy that places emphasis on embodied vocal exploration to expand the client's expressive range, helping them to find their authentic voice and to give voice to that which has been silenced. VMT aims to heal and transform through liberating the voice (acoustic and metaphorical) and freeing the body. It is a very specific way of working with voice and taps into a complex sensory process which connects us to physical sensation, emotional feeling, and our personal narrative, and to archetypes and subpersonalities. Language is inadequate in expressing such multileveled experiences of self; however, vocal sound can. Furthermore, our voice can help us to create meaning, develop self-understanding, and process experiences; to make friends with difficult emotions. VMT is a profound way of reconnecting the bodymind, which brings clarity to habitual breathing patterns, vocal qualities and movement choices, body armour and energy flow – or lack thereof. We learn to notice how intricate and dynamic self-expression really is and how our emotions and history are held in and communicated through our body and voice. Noland (2009) wrote that "the self is the way the self-moves" (p. 168). But the voice is created through physical movement, therefore the self is also how the self sounds. We are body-mind-voice. Identity is created and expressed through movement, image, and voice. Exploiting the overlap between these, VMT provides a lattice as a direct and effective way of working to explore identity and one's sense of self as a lived experience.

A full description of voice movement therapy is outside the scope of this chapter, so I will only elaborate on a few aspects here so that the reader may have an understanding of how I integrate the practice with mask work. I must state that simply including vocal sound when one has a mask covering the face is in no way effective in therapy – or in theatrical performance, for that matter. In fact, for the person in therapy, such practice could lead to further feelings of shame, isolation, and disconnection and is strongly discouraged. The mask that has personal meaning pulls focus on our vulnerabilities – I recommend voice and breath work about the area of personal

DOI: 10.4324/9781003365648-7

exploration prior to incorporating the mask. I also encourage following a slow-paced and mindful donning ritual that allows the gradual integration of mask, movement, breath, and voice. Inviting the voice to emerge on its own without preconceived expectations of sound quality or verbalisations, is a more constructive approach.

The VMT Ten Vocal Components

In VMT, practitioners work with ten vocal components: pitch, pitch fluctuation, glottal engagement, register, volume, vowel, free air, disruption, timbre (flute, clarinet, saxophone), and violin. Each of these components requires a unique movement or physical action within the vocal apparatus and/or body of the "singer" in order to be produced. Each voice is made up more or less of these components and limitations within a component often suggest psychological restriction. Just like a person's emotional state can be read through their movement quality, body language, and posture, VMT practitioners can tune into the psychological and emotional state of a person through their use of the ten vocal components. The sound of the voice reflects the physical and emotional reality of the person and each of these components holds certain aspects of the psyche. In working towards healing, VMT practitioners find ways to support the client in expanding their use of the vocal components and in that way discover and explore aspects of themselves that are perhaps unexpressed or are not allowed to be expressed in other settings or relationships.

VMT as a therapeutic process requires physical action and creative engagement from the client – it is not a passive modality. The healing comes from within the client and, through their intentional physical and vocal crafting of ideas, images, and feelings, they are called to create and evolve new movement repertoires and different ways of performing their identity. VMT shares a way to transform experience out of the very building blocks of identity.

The Mask as Catalyst

The mask works as a catalyst in two primary ways: as an object and as an image. As an object, the donned mask adds weight and a different shape to our head, which influences our musculoskeletal system and how we hold ourselves. The mask also changes our vision, sometimes affects our sense of hearing, and, if we incorporate vocal exploration, the way we sound to ourselves. This brings attention to and challenges our habitual experience of proprioception, interoception, and exteroception, and offers us an opportunity to either play with and investigate a different sense of self, or to hone in and amplify the habitual pattern to better understand it and discover its roots. As an object on the face, the mask demands our full physical engagement and that we place more focus on our body. We slow down and carry ourselves differently to accommodate the mask. The donned mask brings a heightened attention to our face as a surface of communication – because we cannot change the expression of the mask, we must articulate the head, neck, and spine movements more. Often, the first thing we become aware of is a change in breathing pattern. This is a result of the mask on the face but also of the increased levels of charge or anxiety instigated by mask work. In the context of voicework, such physical changes can affect the production and quality of vocal sound. But breathing is tied to emotion and altered breathing can give us information about our state of being. These novel experiences bring a new awareness to self and body and can expand expressive ability in a way that is not possible without the mask.

The mask as an image functions as a trigger to the imagination. As Bakhtin (1984) posits, the mask "rejects conformity to oneself" (p. 40). When we become physically and vocally involved with the image of the mask, our imagination is ignited further. Following and amplifying the imaginings that arrive through creative investigations, we begin to envisage ourselves differently. The mask as image gives us permission to go beyond the mundane habitual self – we can even dislodge ourselves from time, space, and gravity and be something completely different. Mask work demands that the masker is active and creative in the meaning-making process and in the reinvention of the self. Providing the masker with an experience which is incredibly different from their normal repertoire can show them that it is possible to feel different – this gives us something to work towards and to ground in the body as a reference and resource during the transformation process. In this way, it enables the masker to distill personal experience and at the same time raise it to the level of the universal.

As a therapeutic approach, the mask allows us to focus attention on one aspect of self at a time in great detail. As an object and as an image, the mask keeps the masker involved in their process over time. We can use the mask to re-enter the process to continue our investigations. Or we can view the mask as image to reflect, in a very visceral way, on the journey of exploration. The mask is a notable container and transitional object, facilitating the entry into the liminal space of healing and, in its removal from the body, ushering a return to the everyday – although, and importantly, the changes experienced in the masker remain in the body as new neural networks, somatic memory, and body knowledge.

Coming Face to Face with Self: An Autoethnographic Case Study

Since I regard the relationship between masker and mask paramount, I only work with self-made masks that have been cast off the face of the masker.

The initial process of creating a negative face mould and then a positive from which to work is an important threshold into the liminal space of healing that mask work affords. I also work with clay, which, through an embodied and envoiced sculpting process, allows for the specific personally meaningful mask-image to emerge. Integrated from the start and throughout is voice and movement explorations diving deeply into active imagination and awake dreaming. I also collect and create related images, stories, poems, photographs, items, and so on and keep a journal. In this way, I begin to develop the relationship with the mask, and an understanding of this part of the self before the mask has arrived.

When the mask is sculpted, a positive is cast. As soon as it is dry enough to be handled it is placed on the face for the first time through a proper donning process. This is the first real meeting between masker and mask, and time is taken to hold the mask, to look into, breathe, and sing into it and through it – to connect to the mask-as-image and the mask-as-object before placing it on the face. Once donned, I work with breath only and then allow movement to come – there may be some resonance and vocal sound. At first, it is primarily about connecting to how the mask feels on my face and in my body. About paying attention to the soma-sensory system and feeling the differences to one's habitual patterns or the heightening of them. The imagination, active and excited by the mask image and object, then comes into play. Only after some time of curiously following the creative, physical, and vocal impulses, do I look in the mirror, then the exploration is taken deeper, deeper into the body, the voice, and the imagination.

After such initial engagements with the unfinished mask (see Figure 5.1), it becomes clear through the explorations how the mask wants to be aesthetically treated. Throughout this phase, the mask is taken on embodied and envoiced journeys. I incorporate elements that have been collected – for

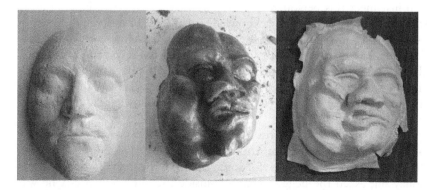

Figure 5.1 Mask creation.
Photographed by the author.

example, images, symbols, poems, dreams, and so on – into the explorations. It is a weaving process that allows image, movement, and voice to knit together. The relationship is consolidated, and this part of the self gains great clarity. Trust in the mask develops and, of course, so does one's trust in self. When the mask is completed, and over time and many courageous journeys of re-engagement, the voice becomes even more clear and specific as the song emerges from the psyche. The movement, posture, and gesture evolve as the body becomes more engaged and alive in *this* expression of self. The narrative around the "character" evolves. The mask is in control, and it begins to reveal its truth and its meaning but only because we are invested and in active collaboration with it. This is not magic. It is a profound and dynamic learning that leads to a new way of experiencing and understanding the self.

The Beggar

When something charges us, makes us uncomfortable, it is often an indication of Shadow. I noticed that I would experience a heightened charge when encountering beggars. I decided to examine this response through investigative mask work. I noticed that when I encountered a beggar, I would avert my gaze to avoid eye contact. I would experience a contraction in my body, a bracing to protect or defend myself. I would feel embarrassed, backed into an ethical corner, and would try my best to leave as soon as possible. I would always say something along the lines of "no, I'm sorry, I don't carry cash." If I was in my car, I would stare forwards willing the traffic light to change to green so I could speed away. So that I could forget this person in need, not have to face their dire situation, their dirty clothes, their failure, their lack of support, and lacking life. And then I would feel guilty for hours afterwards, wondering why I had been such a coward, unable to even just meet this person where they were at. What I was looking away from was myself, refusing to acknowledge that I could easily find myself in just such a circumstance. No one is immune from such a fate; being completely dependent on the charity of others. We are quick to criticize beggars, label them as losers, lazy, addicts, and so on, when in fact we have no idea who they are, what their story and life history is, or what lead them to their situation. But what did this really mean for me and how could I change my habitual response?

In my research I came across Eckhart Tolle's (1999) parable of a beggar (p. 9). The story is of a beggar sitting on the side of the road for many years. One day, he asked a passer-by for some change – the man did not have any money but asked the beggar what was inside the old wooden box he was sitting on. The beggar replied that he did not know but that he presumed nothing. The stranger encouraged him to look inside. On prizing open the old box, the beggar found that it was in fact filled with gold. All this time, the beggar had had exactly what he needed.

This story hit a chord with me. Through my unpacking at the initial research stages of the mask work process, I realized that I had often felt lacking, like I had to beg to be seen, heard, loved, that I was never quite good enough. That I had to live off the scraps tossed aside by others. A feeling of low status, inevitable when one assumes the archetype of the beggar. I noticed that this pattern was part of my sense of self and obviously present in certain relationships. When the archetype manifested itself in me, it had clear physical expression, a collapse in the solar plexus, a sense of shrinking or stooping and skirting around so as not to offend or confront. There were certain vocal qualities too; a lack of clarity in articulation, holding back of sound, and a higher more restricted pitch than normal. In these moments my self-expression was very restricted.

A striking asymmetry emerged as I sculpted the Beggar. The righthand side of the mask became grotesque and inflamed, in excess, fat or puffed out. The left side was drawn in, thin, and hungry. This image spoke to me of excess and lack and that the beggar may paradoxically hold both at once. When the process moved forward into aesthetic treatment, the Beggar needed to be gold (Figure 5.2). When wearing a mask, the masker does not see the outside. The gold represented the value and resources that the beggar doesn't know he has right in front of him. Frequently more obvious to others, we often battle to acknowledge our own gifts and riches.

Whenever I donned the mask and began to embody the beggar, my posture immediately changed – I experienced a collapsing in the solar plexus (a loss of the vertical plane), and a sense of weight came over my body. My muscles felt heavy, drawing off the bone. My breathing became shallow with more force on the short exhalation. My eyesight moved from being focused to being more peripheral. In VMT, the clarinet timbre, peripheral vision, and other aspects of this embodiment indicate a connection with more primal instinctual energy – survival is at the fore. My face drooped, the flesh also giving way to gravity. My tongue became fat. The sound that emerged was lower in pitch than my normal speaking range, the words were not well articulated. There was a thickness about the sound and a whining sometimes, created through the elongation of certain vowels. My voice incorporated some disruption, and a lot of cussing was spewed out with sporadic forceful glottal engagement.

Behind the mask, the face is still active – still expressive, perhaps more so in accepting the invitation of animation. Embodying the subpersonality, the active facial muscles, oral, and suboral cavity allow for different vocal sounds to be produced. The sound quality is affected by the shape of the mouth, lips, tongue placement, the tension or flaccidity of the whole area, and how much of the vocal frequency is moving though the mouth and through

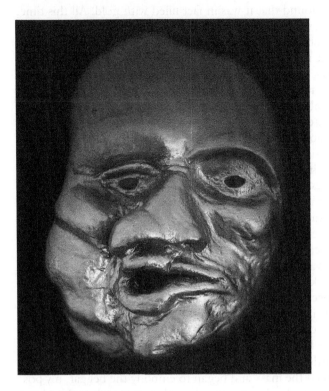

Figure 5.2 Beggar Mask.
Photographed by the author.

the nose and sinus cavity. The quality of sound and my understanding of the emotional and psychological aspects of the VMT ten vocal components allowed a deeper understanding of the archetype, an understanding that is not simply cognitive, but rather an embodied realization. This intricate feeling in the body along with specific vocal vibrations and resonance allow layers of expression and meaning of this part of the self to rise up and travel through the self and the psyche.

Per sona, the sound comes through, perhaps it is the soul that comes through. The Beggar gave permission for the expression of direct, loud, aggressive expressions; the frustrations of not been seen and heard, and not having my needs met came out. Feelings and sounds of deep disappointment and moments that highlighted my habitual repertoire, of recoil and realization that my needs will not be met by the other. I understood the pattern of manipulation, of playing to the other, of giving up on self to appease the other. Feeling the status and levels of power is excruciating, and underlying all of this, the Beggar knows that it is only cruel fate that has created this state. While expressing myself as Beggar, not once did I feel that I had anything of value. I didn't care that I was dirty, and I didn't feel the need to be tidy. As the Beggar, I was closer to a base animalistic part of myself, more instinctual. The Beggar plays a trio with fight and flight and befriend. The body is strung in a state of tension between collapse, readiness to fight, and readiness to run, but at the same time a dire necessity to pander to the other. I became aware of a certain kind of anger that sat in my body. An unexpressed anger that sits just behind the eyes and in the throat. Anger is an emotion I have done a lot of work around, and here was yet another layer calling to be looked at. Mask work never ends, the next image always arrives.

Mask as Mirror: Findings and Reflections

One must face the Shadow to truly know oneself and make progress towards what Jung terms individuation (Jung, 1966). When one works with masks in this way, one literally comes face to face with oneself in a multi-dimensional way. Even after removing the mask, one is left with a tangible embedded memory that can provide a pathway back to the self. The depth of this process always astounds me. I came to a profound understanding of my wound and the relational context of that wound. I realized that, in part, my sense of self and expression of self has been formed around this wound, and realized what parts of myself had been silenced as a result. I realized that my image of self has been carved by all this and how this archetypal energy was at play in my life. I moved from feeling that I was lacking to feeling resourced. The process has anchored in me the knowledge that I have what I need, and I need only to look inside myself to find the gold. Almost ten years later, the process described here still holds, contains, and informs me and continues to teach me about myself and guide me when I'm triggered, when the Beggar comes knocking. Then I recognize my old patterns and I know how to move through and on.

Conclusion

Contrary to the popular opinion of those who lack the courage to truly look at themselves, a mask is not something to hide behind. It is much more useful, more powerful, and more sacred than that! When we enter a meaningful relationship with and a deep acceptance and expression of the part of ourselves that is represented by the mask, we find our soul and a truth that does not leave us. The embodied envoiced mask in therapy has a powerful neurobiological and psychological effect. The active, reflective, and creative experience intentionally amplifies habitual movement and vocal patterns so that they may be examined, explored, and understood on a very visceral level in the present moment. Because it can be removed, the mask can be used to explore and contain Shadow and liminal material, and to explore new ways of being. Of equal importance, working in this way, the client is given permission, and a safe container, to explore new and alternative movement and vocal patterns – even those vastly different from their normal performance of self – thus, the client's expressive ability and imagining of self expands. Embodied and envoiced mask work leads to a new sense of self, the client feels and sounds different, relates differently to others, and is more present in their bodymind and voice while doing so. The envoiced mask in therapy offers a unique way of experiencing self which is not otherwise available.

In an increasingly disembodied world where the truth is hard to come by, working in the flesh and with the truth of sound, movement, and image, we can, in a profound way, come back into harmony with our own personal truth.

References

Bakhtin, M. (1984). *Rabelais and nis world* (H. Iswolsky, Trans.). Indiana University Press.

Jung, C. G. (1966). *Collected works of C. G. Jung* (Vol. 7). Princeton University Press.

Noland, C. (2009). *Agency and embodiment: Performing gestures/producing culture.* Harvard University Press.

Tolle, E. (1999). *The power of now: A guide to spiritual enlightenment.* New World Library.

Part II

Masks at Play

Chapter 6

The Role of Masks in Cultivating Imagination and the Expression of PlayFULLness

Angie Richardson

In a split second, the hesitancy he carries in his body has vanished and he assumes the stance of the creepy, goblin-like creature he has painted on his mask and scampers off into the folds of fabric that delineate his hidey hole...

I have incorporated Māori terms within the text as an acknowledgment of my work in Aotearoa, New Zealand, and the boys, who participated in weekly Creative Arts Therapy sessions, all identify as Māori and are *tangata whenua* (indigenous people) of this land. The four boys (aged ten to 13 years old) attended sessions at their school in Tāmaki Makaurau (Auckland) and, while a flyer had been sent home for their *whānau* (family) explaining what they would be doing, they did not know each other or what was really going to happen. Each boy arrived with his own life story that included adversity and challenges. They presented with a range of psychosocial concerns, including anxiety, low self-esteem, and a seemingly restricted sense of self-identity.

Creative Arts Therapy Group

The overall intentions for the group were to support their emotional and psychological wellbeing, to build confidence in their social relating, and to have some fun! The boys' attendance at the weekly sessions was erratic due to a range of familial situations and school events. This inconsistency made it hard to plan from week to week because of not knowing who would be present at any given time. Although the plan was for 18 sessions over the period of two school terms, it was likely that each boy only attended half that number.

Initially, the framework for the hour-long sessions were ritualised, with a dramatherapy opening and playful warm-up, and then an invitation to engage in visual creative arts-making, and finishing with a ritualized closure.

In the first session, when the boys saw the art table, their eyes lit up as they viewed the materials all laid out in readiness for them. After an

DOI: 10.4324/9781003365648-9

introduction and contributing to a group treaty, outlining agreed behaviors, they engaged in playful non-threatening drama games to get to know each other. Following this, they fell upon the acrylics and brushes as if they had been starved of painting. The resulting artworks showed this may well have been the case, with a couple going right into a state of free form that involved copious amounts of paint flying everywhere! The boys' shared delight in their image-making lessened their nervousness and helped to start connecting them as a group.

The Lead-in Process

The next few sessions followed the pattern of the first, starting with play and drama activities at the beginning and then visual art-making. While one boy was talkative and had a veneer of self-confidence, the others presented as shy, with a couple of them being very quiet and inhibited. Although I felt that art-making was less threatening at this stage than the intensity of immersed dramatic play, I felt that the boys would benefit from an integrative approach. This included different arts materials, providing an opportunity for a sensory experience and agency about what they created, which they seemed to relish. Malchiodi (2015) advocates for an integrative approach when using the expressive arts with children to promote post-traumatic growth. The ritualized dramatherapy interventions offered structure to unknown form, a beginning language for this unfamiliar landscape. This supported a felt sense of safety to encourage the exploration of the spirit of dramatic play, which is a necessary element of spontaneity. Such a framework fits well with Jennings's (2002) take on neuro-dramatic play helping to foster exploratory play while maintaining a safe environment. Jennings also emphasizes the importance of playful attachments for therapeutic work with children who have experienced trauma. A couple of the boys' histories and presentations clearly indicated that trauma was a part of their life experience. As the sessions continued, the boys became more in tune with each other and more willing to be expressive in the drama exercises. As their confidence grew, they became bolder physically and were enthusiastic when the Lycra became a container for what was essentially a tug of war. It was also a means of being physically close together and connecting through laughter.

The warmups encouraged the boys to work together, to listen to each other, and to desensitize them to being looked at by the others in the group (Haen, 2015). These skills are important for being able to have meaningful playful engagement and to support a therapeutic holding space. I believe that this opportunity to develop positively can be missed if there is play deprivation, which is often the fallout from trauma and/or developmentally adverse experiences through challenging life circumstances and an education system that does not fully recognize the importance of teaching and encouraging the art of play.

As the boys became more confident in the space and in being with each other, it was time for a change of scene from art-making to moving into the arena of dramatic play. To encourage dramatic play, the boys were given an option of making huts to play in (Richardson, 2023). As the collection of fabrics tumbled onto the floor, they readily agreed to start creating a *whare* (hut/house) by draping the materials over the tables and chairs. One of the boys seemed more interested in the potential of the fabrics to be used as a costume and he artistically set to work wrapping an ensemble of fabrics around himself, transforming into a character and improvising play as the King (see Figure 6.1).

While this opening phase of the dramatic play was simplistic in nature and continued over a couple of sessions, it laid the groundwork for what was to come. The other three boys occupied the huts and seemed to find it very exciting playing "cat and mouse" with me as I attempted to lure them out from under the fabrics. There was much laughter and energy expelled as the boys crawled and raced about out of reach. While the King quickly claimed his role, the fabrics opened another doorway for him in playing with the notion of instead being a Queen. This energetically charged child-like play helped to strengthen their connections with each other while enjoying the FULL attention of a caring and playFULL adult.

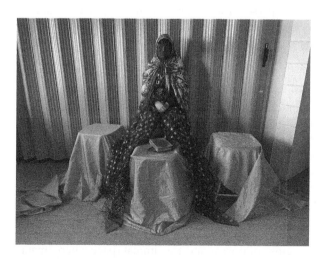

Figure 6.1 **Ruler of the Land.**

Photograph by the author.

Creating the Masks

In week seven, the boys had an opportunity to paint full-faced craft masks that they could use in their dramatic play. As with previous art-making exercises, there was no theme given, no parameters, and they were free to do what they wanted. One of the boys showed a particular intensity with his creation. Previous art-making highlighted an insecure sense of self, as he would be unsure of what to do, unable to come up with his own ideas, and needed a great deal of encouragement to experiment. The mask seemed to call to him and with no hesitation he painted thickly and boldly with one color that had a real intentionality about it. When they were all completed, the satisfaction was palpable even though the finished products could be described as being "modest" in their aesthetics. In essence, they were rough and raw, but there was something about that aesthetic which spoke of authenticity, of being real.

Putting on the Masks

In session eight, all four boys were present and keen to see their masks. After the ritual warm-up, they looked them over and handled them with curiosity, wanting to quickly set up the fabric huts ready for play, then they proceeded to put them on. The masks were now inhabited and suddenly it seemed as if they had sprung to life. The boys immediately melded into the characters their masks called forth, as their entire demeanor changed, including the way they moved their bodies in the space and how they spoke. Their hut preparation also became quite different, with each one having a much more defined space for their own personal *whare*, rather than the shared tunnel-like structures they previously created. Dramatic play ensued spontaneously without any discussion as to who they were or what might happen. While in one respect it was the same scene as before, the masks took it to a whole new level, as the boys' interplay within that ricocheted into something much more complex than a simple game of chase and catch.

Indeed, a more complicated story evolved as the boys explored their characters further, creating four different storylines that segued into one scene. The mask concretized the Ruler of the Land as being a Queen, as s/ he gave orders with a more self-assured theatrical flourish. The other three boys embodied distinctly different characters: a goblin-like creature, a warrior figure, and the attitude and stance of a renegade. This last character almost exaggerated his inner sense of isolation externally by acting out a strong and rebellious persona. My role remained the same – servant to the Ruler. The boys were now immersed in the other realm, that of free-form improvisation under the guise of poiesis and the liminal space where imagination runs freely to be expressed, exercised, and to shape their worldview (Levine, 2015). The boys were fully engaged in embodied dramatic play,

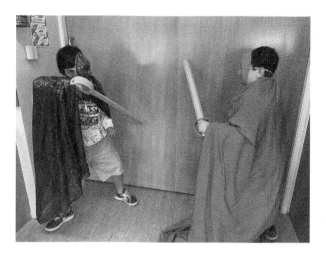

Figure 6.2   Boys in embodied play.

Photograph by the author.

demonstrating that they had the capacity to expand beyond the previously limited playspace (Figure 6.2).

What Followed

Unfortunately, attendance from week eight became quite sporadic for each of them, which hindered a cohesive flow of progression. Certainly, had there been more consistency, it was likely this process would have been even more impactful. However, while the storyline did not particularly develop, there were changes in how the boys interacted during the sessions. In character, dressed in fabrics with the mask on, The Queen became a most graceful and evocative dancer and was visibly elated when the music ended. Another participant, whose history included complex trauma, also underwent quite a transformative journey. While the hut play was extremely helpful in initiating and scaffolding his ability to be playful, the mask was a bridge for him to access some deep internal emotions. Initially, this played out in a contained manner within the group setting; however, in a one-to-one opportunity, he was able to speak into the upsetting *whānau* challenges he was experiencing in his life in a way he had not been able to share before. By the last couple of sessions, it was clear the mask had been a gateway for him to be more fully present in his body and core self. His display of newfound inner confidence was highlighted when he challenged me to a foam sword fight and when he boldly stepped into the role of director, telling his fellow actors how they were to pose for the photos of them in their masks. Just as their

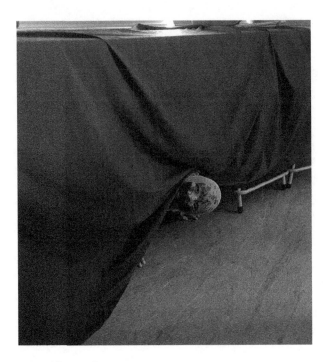

Figure 6.3 The Creature.

Photograph by the author.

newfound characters seemed inspired by their creativity, these interactions extended to interactions without the masks. One member of the group, who was highly anxious, very quiet, and monosyllabic in his verbal interactions, became extraordinarily articulate in his masked character. From the moment he put the mask on, he became delightfully creepy and quite mesmerizing, his character made odd creature-like noises to communicate as he found his voice in a highly creative, unique, and novel way that added to his discovery of a more solid and expansive sense of self (Figure 6.3).

The Role of Relationship and Connection

The lead-up to the mask work was intrinsically important to the therapeutic alchemy that occurred. One of the most important aspects of this *mahi* (work/activity) was developing nurturing and trusting relationships. For *tamariki* (children), who have experienced trauma and/or adversity, the sanctity of the relationship to feel safe is paramount to engaging in a therapeutic process. As Haen (2015) explains, this is a prerequisite for children so "they can step into a process that requires taking emotional and psychological risks that are in opposition to the stifling, self-protective barriers they have established" (p. 239). The quality of the therapeutic relationship with the boys was crucial in creating this safe, bounded space. Levine (1999) wrote about the dynamic relationship in therapy where there is a co-created potential aliveness through the therapist/client relationship. By taking the role of playmate and the good-enough mother, I modeled and encouraged the attitude and skills of being playful through actively engaging in dramatic play alongside the boys. In his book about the connection between play and improvisation, Nachmanovitch (1990) suggests that free, creative improvisation is a vehicle that can facilitate intimacy between players through imaginative play to strengthen friendships in the playspace.

The nature of the sessions was open and organic, following the creative expressive framework, where the emphasis is on nurturing the client's own creative energy to nourish the undeveloped healthy aspects of self (Jennings, 1990). This model highlights the importance of working with the body through movement and sound/voice as a starting place, which was a crucial element of our work before introducing the masks. The neuro-dramatic play model underscores the theories of attachment and play (Jennings, 2002). To this end, the emphasis was on courting the ability to be playful through relationship. For this group, the simpler games such as hut-building and chase-and-catch were crucial building blocks to enable more complex play to evolve.

Delving into the Energetically Charged Realm of the Masks

There was clearly a significance in the boys creating their own masks. While simple in their decoration, there was something that intrinsically connected the boy as maker and the boy as wearer of the mask. Jennings (1990) noted the therapeutic value in having clients create their own masks to wear. She observed how they become absorbed by the creation and, as the creator, the relationship they then have with the mask as the wearer has a shamanic quality, imbued with the spirit of the maker. Mackinnon (2012), a psychotherapist and shamanic practitioner, wrote about the shamanic act of bridging two worlds by crafting an object and comments, "a piece of art is more than a symbol; it is seen as the container of the energy, the very spirit and intent of whatever the object or painting is about" (p. 157). Levine (2015) explores this idea further, by elaborating on the impact of authentic work on both the witness and the creator. The masks did the job of that in a very physical sense by energetically guiding the boys to take on the role that they had in effect unconsciously called forth in an embodied and active state.

Embodiment, Spontaneity, Imagination, and Role/Play Inspired by the Masks

That felt sense of the boys energetically inhabiting the mask was also observable as they became fully embodied in their character. Their body movements were more invigorated and expressive, and they became dramatically creative with their characters' mannerisms and ways of conversing or making sounds. The use of masks therapeutically has transformative qualities of embodied action that provide a novel form of freedom. Roy (2016) felt that the anonymity provided by the mask helps the wearer to literally take up more space with their character's physicality and personality. This liberation can help those who are play deprived, traumatized, and/or overly anxious, who may experience states of "frozen hiatus" in regard to imagination and play. Levine (1999) believes, "The task of therapy...is to mobilize the imagination, to free it up and to loosen the play as much as possible" (p. 260).

The masks were an inroad, a catalyst for the boys to access their imaginations which enticed them deeper into a spirit that engendered fun and novelty and a newfound willingness to be with the unknown. It was here in the unknown playing "in and with" the characters they had called forth where the profound work of growth was nourished (Figure 6.4).

Strikingly, each boy had called forth a character that supported his unique personality and psychosocial needs. The Queen's mask opened the doorway for this participant to role-play with identity and gender. Roy and Ladwig

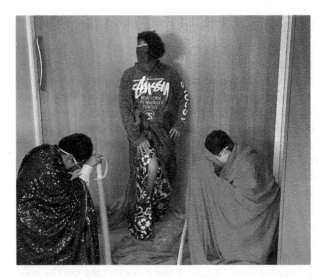

Figure 6.4 Dramatic relationships.
Photograph by the author.

(2015) hypothesize that wearing a mask is a disguise that allows the individual to present a different self, which supports the stage of psychosocial development that Erikson propounds at this age, where children explore who they are. He proposes this stage as the development of identity of self in competition with role confusion. Halprin (2003) suggests that play is an authentic encounter that allows characters to explore emotional territories. For one boy, the mask offered a means to release emotional tension he was carrying using dialectal sound making. In a therapeutic environment, Newham (1999) explains that clients use their voice as a channel to release and express what is going on inside. Several aspects of the masks wove together an opportunity for the boys to play with and strengthen their perception of self. This was readily observable in their ability to engage in authentic interactions in the playspace environment and with one another (Halprin, 2003).

Conclusion

As a creative arts therapist in Aotearoa, I bear witness to intergenerational trauma, a lack of self-worth, loneliness, shame, and fear. *Wairua* (spirit/ soul of a person), life force energy, is "stuck". Often, these children have experienced what is called play deprivation. Pearson (1996) felt that this lost opportunity prevents children from fully exploring aspects of self which can impact them developmentally in later life. Andersen-Warren and Grainger (2000) discussed the necessary role of play being psychoformative, with one purpose of play being to develop the courage to be with what life presents. For those who have experienced trauma or other challenging life events, the creative arts can offer healing in ways that are culturally appropriate and meaningful. This therapeutic journey that these *tamariki* engaged in enabled them to begin reclaiming their innate capacity to be creative and playFULL, more willing to explore and experiment with different possibilities. In this playspace, something intrinsically magical happened when an innocently offered intervention became a potent agent for transformation. When they put on those masks, they had in effect found a powerful dose of soul medicine. My hope would be that this *mahi* helped strengthen their sense of self, so they feel more empowered to shape their own lives positively going forward.

Acknowledgment

I would like to express my *deep aroha* (love, compassion, and respect) and gratitude to these precious *tamariki* for entrusting me to journey alongside them through this unique and soulful experience through dramatic play and for giving me permission to share it in this chapter with their photos.

References

Andersen-Warren, M., & Grainger, R. (2000). *Practical approaches to dramatherapy: The shield of Perseus.* Jessica Kingsley Publishers.

Haen, C. (2015). Vanquishing monsters group drama therapy for treating trauma. In C. A. Malchiodi (Ed.), *Creative interventions with traumatized children* (pp. 3–23). The Guilford Press.

Halprin, D. (2003). *The expressive body in life, art and therapy: Working with movement, metaphor and meaning.* Jessica Kingsley.

Jennings, S. (1990). *Dramatherapy with families, groups and individuals: Waiting in the wings.* Jessica Kingsley Publishers.

Jennings, S. (2002). *Neuro-dramatic-play (NDP) and embodiment-projection-role (EPR).* https://www.suejennings.com/eprndp.html

Levine, E. (1999). On the play ground child psychotherapy and expressive arts therapy. In S. K. Levine & E. G. Levine (Eds.), *Foundations of expressive arts therapy theoretical and clinical perspectives* (pp. 257–273). Jessica Kingsley Publishers.

Levine, S. (2015). The Tao of Poiesis: Expressive arts therapy and Taoist philosophy. *Creative Arts in Education and Therapy, 1*(1), 15–25. https://doi.org/10.15534/CAET/2015/1/4

Mackinnon, C. (2012). *Shamanism and spirituality in therapeutic practice.* Singing Dragon.

Malchiodi, C. A. (2015). Neurobiology, creative interventions, and childhood trauma. In C. A. Malchiodi (Ed.), *Creative interventions with traumatized children* (pp. 3–23). The Guilford Press.

Nachmanovitch, S. (1990). *Free play improvisation in life and art.* Tarcher/Putnam.

Newham, P. (1999). *Using voice and movement in therapy: The practical application of voice movement therapy.* Jessica Kingsley.

Pearson, J. (1996). Child drama: The Peter Slade connection. In J. Pearson (Ed.), *Discovering the self through drama and movement* (pp. 94–103). Jessica Kingsley.

Richardson, A. (2023). How hut making in dramatherapy created a therapeutic play-space. In E. Sweeney (Ed.), *Space, place and dramatherapy: International perspectives* (pp. 29-41). Routledge.

Roy, D. (2016, October 3). Masks as a method: Meyerhold to Mnouchkine. *Cogent Arts and Humanities, 3*(1), 1–11. https://doi.org/10.1080/23311983.2016.1236436

Roy, D., & Ladwig, J. (2015). Identity and the arts: Using drama and masks as a pedagogical tool to support identity development in adolescence. *Creative Education, 6*(10), 907–913. https://doi.org/10.4236/ce.2015.610092

Chapter 7

Mask Work

Increasing Imagination and Developing Self-Awareness in Children: Through a False Face One Finds a True Face

Jhan Groom

Active Imagination

Jung's method of active imagination is an aspect of the "image producing function of the psyche, the imagination" and is at the foundation of mask work (Chodorow, 1997, p. 5). It allows the individual to access the unconscious in waking life and have a dialogue with different parts of the self that live there. This process involves a suspension of rational, critical faculties to "give free rein to the imagination" (p. 6). This results in a working partnership between the conscious and unconscious (Watkins, 1984). Jung believed that the image that appears is an unrecognized, undervalued, or rejected part or attitude of the person creating it. The intuitive use of art materials allows the unconscious to be given physical form because the image arises spontaneously (Chodorow, 1997). Following art making, Jung encouraged his clients to spend time relating to and living with the image through writing and movement exercises, so they could interact with and come to terms with the elements of the unconscious contained in the mask (Chodorow, 1997).

Transformation

The key word to describe the mask and mask work is transformation (Foreman, 2000). The mask is an agent of metamorphosis, changing identity, assuming a new persona, trying out a new way of being, accessing archetypal energy, and traveling to other worlds (Jenkins, 1981; Mack, 1994). The mask acts as a mediator between the individual's conscious and unconscious worlds of the self and is capable of causing a change in character, either through altering how character is represented, or through completely removing the known characteristics of the individual (Keats, 2003). This is done by hiding or modifying the recognizable aspects of the face, which allows the concealed person to present a new or different identity and values. Because the mask conceals the individual's everyday

DOI: 10.4324/9781003365648-10

identity and represents someone or something else, it allows not only a bodily transformation, but behavioral transformation as well, since the wearer's body is "made more expressive by the immobility of the mask" (Johnstone, 1979, p. 204). This process aids the individual's growth by encouraging the individual to experience a broadening of their inner and outer worldview through another being's perceptions, which may lead to an expanded sense of self (Chodorow, 1997). As a result, the individual may have access to energy that contributes to the construction of new cognitions, affect, and behavior, as well as create a new sense of personal control and autonomy, which supports a healthy construction of reality.

The use of masks in therapy provides security for the self, while opening the possibility for the individual to explore multidimensional aspects of their internal world they may not even be aware of, which can result in psychological growth. Masks empower individuals to safely reveal and explore secret thoughts, inhibitions, and attitudes which are usually contained and unexpressed in daily life (Nunley & McCarty, 1999). It is the "disinhibition effect of the mask" that helps individuals to reveal their inner selves, and experiment with new attitudes and behaviors (Janzing, 1998, p. 15). According to Chodorow (1997), psychotherapeutic work with masks gives individuals an externalized symbol of an internal other, which represents a potential agent of change that can result in psychological insight and release of old, outgrown perceptions.

Most therapeutic methods using masks also incorporate the use of art making and drama, which increases the possibility of significant therapeutic change (Chodorow, 1997). Through the experience of dramatizing the mask, the self, mind, and body become better connected, which often results in surprising personal insight.

Children and Masks

Through the usage of metaphor and storytelling, mask making enables a child to look into an inner world and meet a part of themselves they don't know. Behind a mask, the child can safely reveal feelings and emotions not previously recognized or expressed. The mask can help a child express repressed or disguised emotions, depict dilemmas or conflict situations, release personal creativity, assume various forms of identity in a group, explore dreams and imagery, and demonstrate and model different social roles (Boyd Webb, 1991). Working through mask characterization gives the child a broader and deeper awareness and insight into the physical and imaginal self. In this exploration, a part of the child's own personality increases and comes forward to a greater extent than other aspects. The created mask character comes from the individual, yet it is not them (Appel, 1982). It is generally something that is close to the surface of consciousness.

Through this mask work, the creative impulse and instincts of the individual are uncovered, and personal feelings are "unmasked." As a result, the mask wearer is in touch with their own essence, allowing the unconscious and conscious to communicate.

Processing the child's subjective experience of making and wearing a mask is a critical aspect of the masking process (Chodorow, 1997). Because the child, not the mask, is the center of the therapy session, special care, usually in the form of structured activities, needs to be taken in guiding and supporting the child in exploring and constructing the meaning of their experiences. This includes dealing with the active energy of their emotional responses, attempting to try or express new personas, and working out the tensions between the familiar and novel aspects that come up in the masking process (Chodorow, 1997).

Workshop

Client masks that are constructed in therapy should be simple and uncomplicated procedures so they can be created and used in one 75-minute session, or in two 45-minute sessions. If it is being done in two sessions, the first one should contain the mask making and first writing exercise, and the second one the movement and illustration exercises. However, doing the whole process in one session is optimal and preferable. Because it is a quick process, what is revealed will be something close to the surface, and, hopefully, not too difficult to deal with. If an individual engaged in this exercise starts to feel "flooded" or overwhelmed by the feelings coming up or has the feeling the mask is going to "take over," all they need to do is stop, take the mask off, breathe deeply, and relax. Then, in the writing part of the workshop, use that to process the feelings, perhaps even have a dialogue with the mask about what happened, since it is something in them that has a strong need to be expressed. At some point, the individual should put the mask on and complete the process, since the mask character is some part of themselves that needs to be reconciled and accepted. This process can be done repeatedly, since every experience with it will produce a new character to meet, get to know, and integrate.

Materials

Each person is provided a half mask made of posterboard with an attached piece of elastic of about 15 inches. Have available, and spread out over a large area, watercolor paint, brushes, and water containers, felt-tip markers, pencil crayons, colored paper, tissue paper (plain and patterned), curly ribbon, glitter glue, feathers, cotton balls, fake flowers, sparkly paper such as mylar gift wrap, crepe paper streamers, and anything else that can be used to quickly decorate a mask. Also needed will be glue sticks, white glue, staplers, and scissors.

Making the Mask: 20 Minutes

The first 20 minutes are spent in the silent creation of the mask. This is a very intense, intuitive, introspective process, so there isn't any time for chatting, which is also very distracting. Instructions may be given occasionally, or help as needed, and I always call time-markers so people can adjust the pace of their work. Twenty minutes goes by quickly! At the end of the 20 minutes, time is called to end the mask making (Figure 7.1). They must stop whether or not they are finished.

Writing: 7 Minutes

When time is called to end the mask making, the creative materials are cleared away and writing materials are taken out. The individual sits quietly, looks at the mask, letting it "speak" to them. The individual writes five to seven (more, if possible) "I am..." statements from the mask about the mask, such as "I am strong," "I am loving," "I am fierce," etc. They can also use other types of "I..." statements such as, "I fly over tall buildings." If the individual has trouble coming up with "I..." statements about the character of the mask, they can start with descriptive statements, such as "I

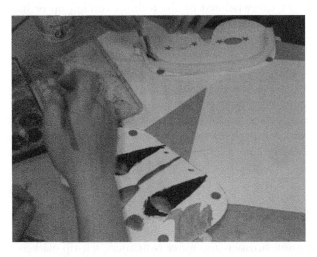

Figure 7.1 Grade-five children intuitively creating posterboard half masks using watercolor paint, stickers, oil pastels, and other art materials.

Photographed by the author.

am green," "I have purple feathers around my eyes," and so on. These statements must be *from* the mask about itself, not from the participant's point of view about the process. I always give a warning a minute before the time ends so they can finish the thought they are working on.

First Exploration

Movement: five to seven minutes; Writing: five to seven minutes

This exploration is all about learning how the mask's body reacts to its environment. Before putting the mask on, the individual is taken through a series of silent movement practices: What does your body do when you are happy? What does your body do when you are angry? Surprised? Excited? And so on. Then the individual is told to close their eyes and put the mask on. When they open their eyes, they are the new mask creature who has never been in this world before and their job is to experience the world through the eyes and body of the mask. How does it move? Fast, slow, heavy, or light? Does it crawl or creep? Is it bold or frightened? The participant explores the environment in which it finds itself. This is done in silence, with no interaction with other masks if this is done in a group. Time is called and the participant goes back to their writing place. Encourage them to keep their mask on as they record, still from the mask character's point of view, what was learned about how the mask's body moved and felt in this new world. A one-minute warning is given so they can finish up the statement they are working on.

Second Exploration

Sound: five to seven minutes; Writing: five to seven minutes

If the individual has taken the mask off, have them close their eyes and put it back on. They assume the body posture of the mask learned in the last movement exercise and move around while they try to find the mask's characteristic sound. This again is without interaction between the mask characters if in a group. They are searching for a sound, not using words, unless they are nonsense words. Is the sound high, low, rough, smooth, melodic, discordant, guttural, nasal? What does it sound like if the character is surprised, happy, scared, angry? What feelings does it create in the body? At the end of the exploration, time is called and they move back to their writing spaces and journals and once again record their findings from an "I" perspective for five minutes. At the end of this, they move on to the next activity.

Illustrating the Character

Drawing: ten minutes; Writing: seven minutes

8.5" x 11" white paper is distributed, and an illustration is done of the character that has been created through the mask work. This is *not* a picture of the mask, but it is an illustration of the character such as would be found with a story in a book. The character should fill most of the page and the illustration can include the setting in which this character lives and acts. It can be drawn with pencil and pencil crayons, felt-tip marker, or paint. It should be in color unless being in black and white is integral to the character and story. When the time to work on the illustration is up, they move to the journaling part of this section, where they record what they have learned about the character through seeing them as a separate entity from the "I" perspective.

Writing the Story and Questionnaire

Now they have 15 minutes to start writing the story of their character (again, from the "I" perspective). This would include background, life, feelings, work, and so on, everything we want to know about someone as we get to know them. This can be in point form to be added to later. As part of the writing and self-awareness aspect of this section, the children are also asked to answer five questions about their experience of the process.

These are the responses of the boy who created the Electric Mouse:

1. *Who or what character came out of your mask?* An electric mouse.
2. *Was this character a surprise? Why?* A little because I had lots of ideas about it.
3. *What do you like/don't like about your character?* It loved to explore/it wasn't that colorful.
4. *How is this character similar/not similar to you?* It's similar because it likes to be adventurous as I am.
5. *What characteristics does this character have that you would like to have/not have?* I don't want to be like him because [he is] evil, scary, and mean.

At the end of 15 minutes for the writing process, the children enter into sharing/debriefing. In a therapeutic session, further discussion would be initiated regarding the characteristics of the mask the child likes, and particularly the ones they don't like. Lois Carey (2006) points out in a case study of a traumatized child that her client's "drawing of the mask developed into enactments of different parts of herself" (p. 62). Where in this child's life does he feel he is "evil, scary, and mean."

Sharing/Debriefing

At this point in the group or individual session, it is good to have sharing and/or debriefing. Participants can share what they learned about their

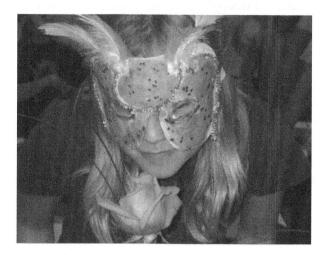

Figure 7.2 The purple and blue feathered mask character of a grade-five student exploring the scent and texture of a rose.

Photographed by the author.

character, show their mask and illustration, talk about their feelings about the character, the process, and so on if they so desire. This is a choice, as for some people, this becomes very personal, and they aren't comfortable speaking about their experience. Encourage them to keep their journals handy to continue to record their thoughts and ideas around this character and process as they continue to develop and come up over the next several days. For further development and insight, the participants can be encouraged to sit with the mask in a quiet place at a quiet time and have a dialogue with it, either verbally or on paper. They can also wear the mask and work with it on their own in front of the mirror to continue to get to know the character better (Figure 7.2). If they desire to take the process further, they could also make a more detailed full-face mask of the character that came out of their illustration and continue their explorations through working with that mask.

Conclusion

Mask making and mask wearing can be used by the expressive arts therapist through the vehicle of active imagination as a creative and effective psychotherapeutic intervention for change, particularly for children. The use of intuitive mask making using a wide variety of art and craft materials, combined with movement and writing exercises, externalizes unconscious material that the creation of the mask brings forward. This allows a hidden aspect of the child, and the feelings associated with it, to be revealed, acknowledged, and experienced through active engagement with the personality embodied by the mask. Troublesome emotions or behavior can be identified, clarified, and solidified through the experience of writing about and illustrating the resulting character. The use of mask work as a therapeutic protocol in a creative and controlled environment ultimately permits children (and adults) to experience connectedness between body and psyche, conscious and unconscious, with the resulting integration of that knowledge contributing to psychological and behavioral growth.

References

Appel, L. (1982). *Mask characterization: An acting process.* Southern Illinois University Press.

Boyd Webb, N. (Ed.). (1991). *Play therapy with children in crisis: A casebook for practitioners.* The Guilford Press.

Carey, L. (Ed.). (2006). *Expressive and creative methods for trauma survivors.* Jessica Kingsley Publishers.

Chodorow, J. (1997). *Jung on active imagination.* Princeton University Press.

Foreman, J. (2000). *Maskwork.* The Lutterworth Press.

Janzing, H. (1998). The use of the mask in psychotherapy. *The Arts in Psychotherapy,* *25*(3), 151–157. https://doi.org/10.1016/S0197-4556(98)00012-4

Jenkins, R. (1981). Two way mirrors. In D. M. Dooling (Ed.), *Parabola: Myth and the quest for meaning* (pp. 17–21). The Society for the Study of Myth and Tradition.

Johnstone, K. (1979). *Impro: Improvisation and the theatre.* Routledge Theatre Arts Book.

Keats, P. (2003). Constructing the masks of the self in therapy. *Constructivism in the Human Sciences,* *8*(1), 105–124. https://search.proquest.com/docview/204586492?pq-origsite=gscholar

Mack, J. (1994). *Masks and the art of expression.* Harry N. Abrams Inc.

Nunley, J., & McCarty, C. (1999). *Masks: The faces of culture.* Harry N. Abrams Inc.

Watkins, M. (1984). *Waking dreams.* Spring Publications Inc.

Chapter 8

Using Neutral Masks with Adolescents

Tsufit Shemer

Masks have been used in various fields, such as rituals, shows, and theater performances, as well as in various types of therapy, including art therapy. The neutral mask creates a visual image of an expressionless human face. The uniqueness of the neutral mask is its lack of specific characterization, which creates a generalized human. Out of neutrality grows the possibility to express and embody any emotion, any identity, any character, any gender, and any status. In 1960, the director Jacques Lecoq used the neutral mask as a training tool for acting students. By working with the neutral mask, students practice a neutral state as performers. They become a *tabula rasa* (a blank slate). According to Lecoq (2000), the neutral mask allows the performer to reach a state of mental and physical awareness, to be present in the moment. The neutral state is a primary starting point of awareness and intention. According to Eldredge and Huston (1978), "The mask helps to identify a resting state for the actor, a condition of presence from which all things are possible" (p. 28). The neutral mask hides the entire face. Working with the mask emphasizes physical expression, as opposed to the usual means of communication, such as voice, words, and facial expressions. The color of the mask depends on the material from which it was made. Neutral masks used to train actors are usually made of leather, papiermâché, or Celastic (plastic-infused fabric that becomes moldable when activated by a solvent).

The Mask as a Therapeutic Tool in Art Therapy

In therapy, the mask is an image of the self. It is used as a projective technique to separate one part of the self from another (Landy, 1985). The mask simultaneously hides and reveals the person wearing it. It conceals and hides the individual face, and reveals his behavior, movement, gestures, and more (Eldredge & Huston, 1978). Steinhardt (1992) claimed that working with masks allows patients to connect to their strengths. With the help of the mask, the patient becomes a screenwriter, a director, and an actor

DOI: 10.4324/9781003365648-11

at the same time. The mask expresses a character that already exists in the individual in one way or another.

Landy (1985) distinguished between three approaches for using masks in therapy. The first is more distant. The individual plays with the masks spontaneously and creates some kind of story. The story can reflect a personal experience, or it can be distanced by reference to the characters in the third person or in a "once upon a time" framework. In the second approach, the individual works with the mask, assuming roles of the family characters, and engaging in dialogue with other characters. The third approach is psychodramatic. The therapist, or other group members, play auxiliary ego roles, such as mother, father, sibling, or self. The individual's dilemmas can be brought into focus through a confrontation with the auxiliary ego.

Jones (1996) referred to the mask as a projection object. He indicated three main points regarding dramatic projection when working with masks. First, the form of the mask affects the content that is projected. Second, with the help of the mask, individuals express parts of their personality that were denied or hidden and attribute these to the mask and not to themselves. Third, the mask allows focusing and presenting certain aspects or parts of the self.

Group Drama Therapy

This chapter describes the creation of neutral masks by young adolescents who attended group drama therapy sessions in middle school in Israel. The groups are held during school hours. Session length is 45 minutes. The counselor and sometimes the school psychologist do an initial screening of the students who can benefit from drama group therapy. The group meets in a therapy room at the school. In the treatment room, there is a table and chairs, a rack with costumes and various accessories such as glasses and hats. In the closets of the room, there are board games and playing cards, a soft ball, and various art materials. The group meets once a week throughout the school year, from September or October to June. At the beginning of the meetings, there is a short pulse around in which everyone tells how they feel. In the rest of the meeting, each participant chooses what he wants to do. In each group, as the year progresses, a repertoire of games and activities is formed that the participants choose again and again. The groups referred to in this article included the same participants throughout the year.

A Wounded Mask

Aron is a 12-year-old boy who is albino and visually impaired (due to sensitivity to sunlight). Aron's parents describe him as a victim of social rejection due to his appearance. His albinism and visual impairment are not discussed at home. He lives with his parents and older sister. Aron was diagnosed with mild attention deficit disorder, with an emotional basis. His parents insisted that he study in a class for students with learning disabilities.

Aron came to group drama therapy with two other students from his class. It was their first year in this middle school, after six years in different elementary schools. Each of the participants faced social difficulties in school. The goal of the group was to develop their social skills and provide a space where they could share their various difficulties and process the transition from elementary school to middle school. At the beginning of the year, the group discussed the experience of social rejection, which all the participants went through at one time or another. The therapy continued throughout the school year.

Aron almost never spoke explicitly about his social and physical difficulties. He seemed happy to come to the group meetings and sought interaction and joint play with the group members and with me. Aron often verbally teased the other group members, possibly out of a desire for attention and interaction with them. They did not tease him back; while the other two group members became closer during the year, Aron's social place in the group and his class remained the same.

The participants mostly engaged in dramatic play. Aron often played a shrewd and powerful bandit, while another group member was the *schlemiel* (misfit) and unsuccessful bandit. The third participant and I played the victims, ordinary people who were being robbed in a bank, café, or store. Aron had various ideas for the course of the drama and the development of the plot. Sometimes the robber he played would escape, and other times he was caught by the police.

Creating the Mask

During one meeting, one of the participants was looking for the neutral mask that had been used for the bandit character in the group dramatic play. In the supply cabinet, he found a package of neutral masks and asked if he could paint one of them. Aron joined his request. The neutral masks were made of white plastic. The inside is smooth, and the outer part has a rough texture, like velvety fabric. This allows for the use of a variety of art materials such as markers, watercolors, acrylic paint, and more.

Aron put a mask on a table, sat down, chose markers, and began to draw on the mask (Figure 8.1). He seemed to be concentrating and did not speak to the other members of the group, which was not typical for him. He chose a black marker and a dark green marker. He drew two thick lines from the upper edge of the mask, each line with a different marker. The lines formed a hollow rectangle around the forehead area and to the lower end of the nose. He colored in the rectangle with a yellow marker. He then chose a red marker and colored around one of the eyes, down the cheek, and under the

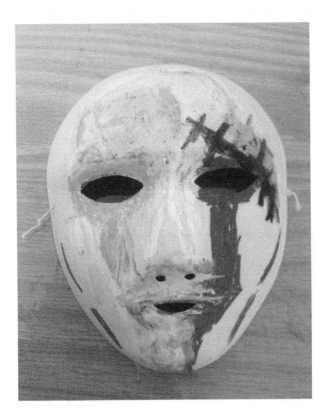

Figure 8.1 Aron's mask.

Photographed by the author.

nose and mouth. Aron looked at his mask and said, with enthusiasm, "His brain is spilling out and dripping down his face."

He paused, looked at the mask, and studied it for a few moments. Then he asked me if I had correction fluid because he wanted to erase some things from the mask. I gave him a bottle of correction fluid, and he erased the rectangle and the lines he had drawn. The correction fluid didn't erase the lines as Aron wanted, so I suggested that he use white oil pastel. With the white oil pastel, he colored over the red part he had drawn. He explained that he wanted to "make it a scar" and for it to look like an "old wound." He highlighted the area around the eye with pink oil pastel. When he finished, he tried on the mask. Aron continued to work on the mask during several more sessions. In one meeting, he added a black scar above one eye. In another meeting, he drew a red spot around and below the other eye, with red lines along the sides of the mask. He said that these were scars. After finishing his work on the mask, Aron would wear it when he played the character of a strong and menacing bandit.

Summary and Reflection

The neutral white mask, like a blank page, can be thrown and drawn on with different colors, materials, and textures. It has limits but is full of possibilities. Kandinsky (1911/1977) saw the color white as a color of deep silence and primary formation – the creation. Netzer (2008) stated that white is seen as purity, innocence, and holiness, but also death since paleness is associated with a lack of energy. Netzer claimed that there is universality in the symbolism of colors, alongside cultural variation and personal meaning. While white is associated with purity and spirituality in our culture, we also perceive albinos as abnormal, strange, and even sick. The mask is an inanimate plastic work of art that stands on its own, as a creation of a character with certain traits that will come to life and be acted out.

Aron, who did not talk about his personal difficulties and avoided openly dealing with his disabilities, often chose to play the role of the strong, shrewd, and menacing bandit in the drama, and he created a mask with bruises and wounds, battle-hardened and representing great pain. The bandit he played was busy threatening and stealing, taking from others, as an attempt to fulfill his needs. Through his choice to embody a strong, powerful, and threatening character, he revealed his pain, fear, weakness, and ability to survive.

The wounds that Aron created and which he went over again and again with the white oil pastel turned into scars, as if time had passed and the wounds had healed, but a memory of what happened remained. Aron created a layered representation of his painful experience, in which there was interplay between the visible and the hidden. It was no longer possible to make out all the first lines that Aron drew on the mask. Is it possible to erase pain? Do emotional experiences leave scars? Creating the mask, playing with it, and embodying the character of the bandit while wearing it allowed Aron to deal with emotional content in a nonverbal way. By using the mask, which was a visual expression of inner feelings, Aron took off, for a few minutes, the "mask" that he wore every day.

A Mask with Worms

Ben is a 13-year-old boy. His father died when he was six. He lives with his mother and her partner. Ben has an older sister who does not live at home. He had learning disabilities at preschool and verbal and emotional difficulties. In elementary school, he occasionally hit other children out of frustration at being unable to express himself. He suffered from social rejection and bullying. As an adolescent, Ben has difficulty initiating and maintaining social relationships. His mother said that he often locks himself in his room and plays computer games.

Ben came to group drama therapy with three other students, each from a different class in the same grade. The purpose of the group was to develop their social skills and abilities. The therapy continued throughout the school year. Ben was very withdrawn in the group meetings throughout the process. He avoided sharing personal experiences. When there was a round in which everyone spoke about how they were doing or different experiences they had the previous week, Ben would briefly answer with a word or two, but no more. Sometimes he would cooperate with games I initiated, but for the most part, he refused. As the therapeutic process progressed, Ben connected with one participant in particular – Joey. They played ball and board games together. Their interaction showed other sides of Ben: playfulness, energy, humor, and a desire for friendship. Their relationship continued even outside the weekly group meetings.

Creating the Mask

In the beginning of the group process, it was difficult to gather the four participants together around a joint activity for any length of time. In one of these meetings, Ben and Joey saw neutral masks in the supply closet in the studio and wanted to paint them. They sat together and began to draw. Ben, who was very passive in the group, seemed focused and active. He worked quickly, thoroughly, and with great skill. Using pink plasticine, he created a wound on the forehead and three-dimensional thick worms crawling in and out of the mask. Ben used a glue gun to make holes in the plasticine worms and added drops of hot glue on the mask. He seemed to be familiar with using various materials. While working, he turned to me and enthusiastically showed me the mask during various stages of work. He put on the mask and asked me to take his picture. Toward the end of the meeting, Ben and Joey had fun together, wearing the masks they made and some hats that were on the props rack. Ben continued to work on the mask in subsequent meetings. He added red color by melting a red oil pastel with the hot glue gun and added blue marker marks (Figure 8.2). After he completed the mask, he put on the mask again, took it off after a few moments, and did not use it anymore.

Summary and Reflection

Ben, who seemed introverted, quiet, and sometimes disconnected from the group activity, became full of life, creativity, pleasure, and satisfaction while working on the mask. During the creation process, Ben revealed abilities and skills that he had not shown before. The neutral mask is a platform for projection. It enables the expression of issues and experiences that are

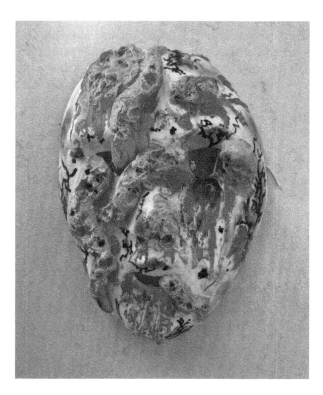

Figure 8.2 Ben's mask.

Photographed by the author.

difficult to voice in words. Steinhardt (1992) said that creating and looking at a mask allows for an internal dialogue with silenced and hidden parts of oneself. Images, feelings, desires, and fears are embedded in the mask. It seems that, through the mask, Ben revealed his experiences of vulnerability, horror, rejection, and disgust. He did not reveal these issues to the group in any other way during the therapy process.

As Levine (1992) wrote, the purpose of therapy is to express pain and suffering, to embody the pain, rather than eliminate it: "Expression is itself transformation… This is the message that art brings" (p. 14). The mask, then, is a tangible expression and embodiment of pain. Ben was possibly showing the pain of rejection, loss, vulnerability, loneliness, and transitional difficulties. It seems that the mask carried these feelings during the meetings in which Ben worked on it. While creating the mask, he behaved in a more relaxed and communicative manner. The connection that he developed with Joey while creating the mask led to a friendship that continued outside the therapy room.

Conclusion

This chapter briefly described using neutral masks in dramatherapy with adolescents who had experienced bullying, rejection, and abandonment. They used various art materials to create layers of cuts, wounds, and scars on the masks as an expression of their pain. The mask is an intermediary between the inside and outside, the actual and fictional, covering and revealing. In a mask, we remain ourselves, yet also become someone else. The power of the mask lies in its possibility to unmask parts of the self, carrying the internal and external together. The mask provides a measure of distance for the maker, who can attribute parts of their personality that had been denied to the mask and not to themselves. This distance is especially important in therapeutic work with adolescents, who often resist direct contact with personal experiences and emotional exposure.

References

Eldredge, S.A., & Huston, H.W. (1978). Actor training in the neutral mask. *The Drama Review*, 22(4), 19–28. https://doi.org/10.2307/3181722

Jones, P. (1996). *Drama as therapy: Theatre as living*. Brunner-Routledge.

Landy, R. (1985). The image of the mask: Implications for theatre and therapy. *Journal of Mental Imagery*, 9(4), 43–56. https://www.researchgate.net/publication/232419248

Lecoq, J. (2000). *The moving body*. Bloomsbury Methuen Drama.

Levine, S. K. (1992). *Poiesis: The language of the psychology and the speech of the soul*. Palmerston Press.

Netzer, R. (2008). *The magician, the fool and the empress: The tarot cards in the cycle of life and in therapy*. Modan Publishing House.

Steinhardt, L. (1992). Hidden and visible: Masks as a therapeutic tool. *Journal of YAHAT- the Israeli Association for Creative Arts Therapies*, 1(1), 23–30. https://ajcat.haifa.ac.il/index.php/en/about

Chapter 9

Victim Empathy

Unmasking Vulnerability

Nancy Jo Cardillo

Out of the social consciousness of the 1960s, the experience of victims and their rights became a priority of the criminal justice system due to a rise in crime (Office for Victims of Crime, 2005). In 1972, correctional institutions across the Western world designed victim empathy programs and assessment protocol facilitating the field of victimology . The Massachusetts Department of Youth Services (DYS, n.d.) is one program providing clinical and rehabilitative services. The material here draws from an expressive arts therapy (EAT) empathy group in a Massachusetts maximum secure treatment facility serving youthful offenders. Initiated by an art therapist (AT) at Raw Art Works (n. d,), the group was taken on by a dance/movement therapist (DMT).

Victim Empathy

Empathy is considered an essential character trait for morally just societies, providing harmony, personal growth, and thriving, reciprocal relationships. Disruptive, anti-social behavior in childhood is linked to weakened empathy and later criminal activity (Hunnikin et al., 2020). From infancy, empathy should be addressed throughout life (Stern et al., 2021; Trivedi-Bateman & Crook, 2022). Cultivating empathy in the criminal justice system, however, is a complex psychological process that is easier said than done. Without empathy, an individual is unable to fully attend to others or gauge right from wrong (Potter, 2004). It enables adolescents to make sense out of difficult situations and coinciding emotions about the conflict and the individuals involved. Adolescent responses are often situation-specific. Situational reinforcers, such as substance abuse and other risky behaviors, peak during this stage of identity exploration (Coetzee, 2020). Empathy can play a big part in moral reasoning and relevant behaviors, potentially returning youth to their own moral code (Malti et al., 2012) .

Victim empathy is defined as "the offender's understanding of the victim's pain or the impact of his offenses" (Carich et al., 2003, p. 257). It

DOI: 10.4324/9781003365648-12

requires the ability to read another's body language: facial expression, vocal intonation, posture, and gesture. Known as "victim personalization," the goal is to develop empathy for one's victim until it becomes reflexive, extending to other potential victims . Remorse for harming another comes gradually, requiring a safe space to work through denial, assume responsibility, and face one's history as a victim (Smith, 2017). The empathy group capitalized on opportunities to facilitate empathy, creating a "we-centric space" (Gallese, 2009, p. 520) – changing the DNA of the moment.

The Empathy Group – DYS Facility

The empathy group met in the designated art space: a cramped basement with barricaded windows. Participants identified as females, aged 13 to 17 years old. Their sentences were determined by their crimes, which included acts or threats of bodily harm, car thefts resulting in injury or death, armed robbery, and shootings. All services, including educational, recreational, and clinical, took place behind bars. Whenever leaving the facility, residents were handcuffed and possibly shackled. Youths with open cases were held in uncertainty, lengthening their stay potentially for years.

Considering the many histories of sustained abandonment, abuse, and violence, the question became how the body self-concept of these girls might affect their empathic ability? Research indicates that even adolescents lacking secure family relationships can catch up in empathic care behaviors. Stern et al. (2021) suggest that group programs which model empathy and incorporate "reflective discussion" elicit a "felt sense of security," helping youth internalize empathic behavior (p. e1338).

Shifting the focus from AT to DMT, activities were reworked through the lens of the body via the practice of kinesthetic empathy and attachment theory. The movements involved in the shared roles of mask making became an instrument of kinesthetic empathy – "the embodiment of empathic processing" (Berrol, 2006, p. 308) – which depends on motor representations in the brain (Gallese, 2009; Rizzolatti et al., 2002). This duet and the choreography of empathy are the focus of this writing (Foster, 2011).

Besides the guard, the six girls in the group were chosen by personality, essential to any group's success, especially so in a correctional facility. The group's viability depended on diversity. A mixture of quiet and outgoing individuals created a group dynamic allowing varied expressive styles to learn from and *feel into* each other's experience. According to Carich et al. (2003), when addressing victim empathy, "The ideal group environment involves vulnerability, support, cohesion, and compassion, and includes 6 to 12 group members" (p. 265). To this, add humor!

In DYS settings where youth live together and are deprived of basic amenities and freedoms, vulnerabilities are preyed upon, defenses are challenged, competition and insults surface, and cliques form. Before cohesion was achieved, razzing was frequent and could abruptly escalate. In worse case scenarios, offenders were removed by guards preventing the DMT from completing the curative steps towards resolution and repair. So, if teaching empathy to incarcerated girls might make a positive difference in behaviors, but the girls are acting out before they can learn this, then the question became, "how can the groups be amended so each participant can benefit?"

The First Group Meeting

In the first group, introductions led to co-creating community agreements. The DMT started by asking some basic questions: What is empathy? Are we born with empathy? Can empathy be learned? Everyone received paper and markers to quickly sketch a variety of feelings. This got them out of their heads, expanded their expressive repertoire, noted interpersonal similarities and differences, and established a schema distinct from their other groups.

There are other techniques that foster victim empathy: readings and films portraying victim impact; letters written to victims (typically not sent); victim impact collages; role play; responding to victim questions, such as, "Why me?" (Carich et al., 2003, p. 267). Smith (2017) added psychodrama's empty chair technique. In this empathy group, prior to mask making, the DMT presented activities to build empathy, including lifeline drawings – a single line taken into movement. Using the prompt, "In the safety of my home, a child will have...," participants delved into their personal stories by creating dioramas using images from children's books. In response to the film, *Once Were Warriors* (Scholes, 1994), they collaged the heart of someone they struggled or identified with. They decorated a shoe, conveying what it takes to walk in their shoes. It was touching to see how many girls picked baby shoes out of the pile. Could this be a metaphor for the longings of an inner child or a lost soul?

Given the trauma history in the room, the DMT offered comments to dissuade youth from avoiding painful feelings or transferring their personal pain into anger towards another. These conversations modeled the importance of having compassion for one's own troubling past, opening empathy for another by first feeling empathy for oneself.

Perhaps for the first time, the girls were encouraged to sit with the sensations and feelings that they held towards their creative work, as well as the group's responses to them. Despite being in prison and under strict surveillance, the girls began to recognize that the boundaries of expression – what they could or could not say, do, and show – were different here than elsewhere in their day-to-day reality. The tenor of the empathy group's emphasis on exploration, originality, kindness, and acceptance was freeing for some, and, at the very least, a "form" of freedom for others.

Preparing the Group for Mask Making

When former participants displayed their decorated masks, others took notice and wanted one, too. This highlighted the deprivation of and longing for things of beauty and spirit. Each girl saw herself reflected in her self-made mask. This speaks to how nurturing the materials themselves can be. In the words of Bread and Puppet (1984), "ART IS FOOD. You can't EAT it BUT it FEEDS you."

Mask making is a partner activity with joint vulnerability. The receiver surrenders control, with eyes and mouth closed, while their partner must be trusted to mindfully apply the mask materials in a safe way. In preparation, the following guidelines were discussed and demonstrated:

- Touch is required.
- The one applying the mask must always maintain physical and verbal contact with the partner who has their eyes closed.
- If the person who is applying the mask needs to leave their partner's side, they will ensure their partner's comfort by requesting the therapist to replace them.
- Be sensitive! The receiver needs to breathe! Be careful when covering the eyes, nose, and mouth with plaster strips and ensure openings at the nostrils.
- Layer the strips, gently smoothing rough edges.
- When the mask hardens, tell the therapist.
- When all three masks are ready, the group witnesses each receiver as they take off their mask and view it for the first time.

Therefore, mask making for incarcerated youth was an exercise in bravery for some and trust for all. Participants came into the project pre-wired for issues to come up. The active-passive nature of mask making and the vulnerability of surrendering control, of being touched, of someone leaning in close – breath to breath, body to body – was a big risk. An earlier guided imagery exercise and the sharing afterwards revealed that some participants, due to their histories, tended to seek refuge in sexual fantasies. This, too, needed to be considered when preparing the youth for the intimacy of the mask making process. Therapists need to be watchful for signs of fight-or-flight. As noted by Panda et al. (2021), these are "all issues that require compassionate care from providers" (p. 2).

Mask Making: An Empathic Duet

Once the guidelines were understood, participants were ready to engage their curiosity. A buffet of photographs showing masks from different cultures was presented to them. These masks, from the practical to the fantastical, were created for purposes such as protection, religion, healing, theater, identity, sport, and more. The masks that the girls created were constructed from plaster cloth, which had been pre-cut into strips. The strips were then dipped into water and smoothed onto the face. Participants who were concerned about having their entire face covered had the option to create a half mask or to leave their eyes uncovered. Those who could not tolerate touching or being in close proximity with another person were offered the option of being part of the "safety patrol." Walking the room, they monitored the stress levels of their peers, and replenished materials as needed. These various options allowed participants a sense of control.

Despite the studio's drab visage, ambient music played to support a sense of self-care and wellbeing. Once partnered, the person applying the mask set up their "station" with water and plaster strips, much like a manicurist with a client. Their partner spread Vaseline on their own face to protect their skin and make it easier to remove the mask when dry. From this point on, the girls agreed to stay with each other until both masks were complete. Now sitting side by side, partners took turns to give and receive the cloth strips.

Consider for a moment the inner landscape of the reclining and receiving partner. Again, the earlier guided imagery exercise to prepare participants for this activity was a crucial step, given the background histories of this population. As the mask progresses, more skin is touched, including erogenous zones such as lips, eyelids, eyebrows, and temples. Slowly, eyes are completely covered. This experience might bring up traumatic sensations, memories, images, thoughts, or feelings. The youth might feel mounting panic, visualize a hand over their mouth, or think "I can't scream!" A mask applied to one's face could trigger claustrophobia, such as thoughts of being trapped or even locked-up.

It's critical to note that participants were never helpless and could stop the process at any point.

No girl experienced heightened trauma during this activity, the last in the eight-to-ten-week program, due to the level of trust previously achieved. When working with victims of sexual exploitation and/or physical abuse, clearly, the therapist needs to be vigilant.

For the partner applying the mask, this was their chance to assume a role in the prison (or life, perhaps) that was not often asked of them. By the nature of the assignment, and the purposeful role of "mask maker," they became a protector and nurturer. Internal and external stereotypes such as "hormonal teenager," "juvenile delinquent," or "violent criminal" were pushed aside, and the mask maker had an opportunity to redress these labels and portray another aspect of their being.

In other words, to mold the mask, they had to gently touch another person's face separately from any trauma and intuitively respond to their verbal and nonverbal cues. Doing so, they expanded their affective and relational vocabulary, as supported by neuroscientific research linking perception with touch. Keysers et al. (2010) observed a somatosensory dimension to the empathic understanding of others, strengthening the colloquial notion "that other people's sensations, pain and actions can be touching" (p. 417).

Unmasking Vulnerability

Finally, the plaster mask was hardened enough to be lifted off the skin. Each girl had endured a tedious process leading to this pivotal moment, ending the quiet waiting and wondering. The first glimpse was nothing short of poetic, such was the feeling of awe when witnessing the transformation that unfolded as each recipient viewed their "face" in their hands for the first time. These youth, who had endured such traumatic experiences, often beyond their control, were skilled at finding ways to not "look" at themselves. Now, they were looking through empathic lenses and uncovering an aspect of self that had perhaps never been "seen." A mask invites a new spirit into the room, for it "enacts a dialogue between...the exterior and the interior, the seen and unseen" (Pennick, 2022, p. 1). There was respect and a reprieve found in the vulnerability, innocence, and grace of that moment.

The mask became evidence of a mutually caring act, of a generous offering of time, concentration, and positivity. The girls held their masks in their purest, simplest, most raw state, unpainted and unadorned, while the DMT allowed a quiet time for the range of emotions.

It's worth noting that, unlike the distorted viewing of oneself in mirrors, photographs, or on Zoom, the mask permits the recipient to see their face in three dimensions, the way others perceive them. Since masks were talked about as transformative during the warm-up, the DMT repeated the aspect of the mask being transformative; representative of new beginnings and change – a chance to see oneself as unblemished and unmarked.

Finishing Touches

For many participants of the empathy group, the concrete task of decorating their mask was the moment they were waiting for. For the DMT, the empathic process had already taken place in the kinesthetic and tactile dance of give-and-take described above. Agreeing with Richardson (2022), the exploration of materials "parallels exploring the emotional content of imagery" (p. 130). Creativity is "a spiritual path in its own right," according to Pennick (2022), author of *The Spiritual Power of Masks: Doorways to Realms Unseen* (p. 4).

Decorating the mask then became important for continued self-attunement, representation, and identity formation. Participants were presented with an array of household and natural materials (sandpaper, Band-Aids, mesh, petals, feathers) as well as craft items. Painting symbols of racial and gender pride, gluing on teardrops, and portraying a safe, innocent, sleeping self were frequent motifs. Later, improvisational movement and writing prompts were offered to bring story to their masks.

Relational Repertoire and Summary

Close proximity in a detention facility does not always lead to a negative, reactive, or intrusive experience. While constructing their masks, if partners perceive their environment supportively, then instead of distress or fear of harm or rejection, the "being with" could elicit a shared understanding. Irrespective of their prior connection to each other, integration can develop from an emotion generated by the positive interpersonal exchange (Montoya et al., 2018).

Intra- and interpersonal trust, empathy, and an attachment-secure state of mind (Stern et al., 2021) were the desired outcomes for this empathy group. The mask became a safety valve and intermediary boundary. It enabled the giver and the receiver to explore less familiar parts of themselves with the knowledge that an adult (DMT/EAT) was there to watch over them, offering protection; most likely not the case at the time of any previous trauma.

A core principle of DMT states that to expand an individual's movement repertoire is to expand their options for relating (Leventhal, 2012). The active-passive, nonverbal postures and gestures required to make a mask, such as leaning in, eye contact, gentle touch, attunement, and reciprocity, are "emotion-specific behaviors" (Montoya et al., 2018, p. 675). This is associated with Western interpretations of interpersonal trust and has the potential to reformulate one's relational body self-image. According to Sheets-Johnstone (2010), paying attention to one's own movement leads to a sense of self-agency, which Leventhal (2012) elucidates can contribute to an expanded perceptual focus and increased awareness of options and choices so important to youthful offenders.

The body is a container storing life's experiences, and each time a positive experience is added – especially when witnessed through a shared trust – it becomes part of the inner, healing fabric of the individual. Mask making encompasses the neurophysiological experience of oneself as an empathic being. Since mirror neurons (the neural basis for empathy) engage more readily with the familiar (Calvo-Merino et al., 2005), the repetitious application, anticipation, and turn-taking in making a mask extend the brain's range, integrating the cognitive, affective, *and* bodily facets of empathy. This enables the unfamiliar to become familiar, creating a suitable laboratory for empathy.

The process of crafting a mask strengthened the DYS's goal of developing "pro-social" skills towards victim empathy. For the DMT, "pro-social" translated into the girls becoming their own agents: *My body-self as capable of setting boundaries, of being expressive, lovable, caring, and ready to make wise choices today and onward into the future.*

This chapter is dedicated to the memory of Beau Diehl, art therapist and mentor who embodied the meaning and movements of empathy.

References

Berrol, C. (2006). Neuroscience meets dance/movement therapy: Mirror neurons, the therapeutic process and empathy. *The Arts in Psychotherapy, 33*(4), 302–315. https://doi.org/10.1016/j.aip.2006.04.001

Bread & Puppet. (1984). Why cheap art manifesto. https://1284bf722a.nxcli.net/cheap-art/why-cheap-art-manifesto?_ga=2.18522297.1621731534.1669935953-92124877.1669935953

Calvo-Merino, B., Glaser, D. E., Grèzes, J., Passingham, R. E., & Haggard, P. (2005, August). Action observation and acquired motor skills: An fMRI study with expert dancers. *Cerebral Cortex, 15*(8), 1243–1249. https://doi.org/10.1093/cercor/bhi007

Carich, M., Metzger, C., Baig, M. S. A., & Harper, J. J. (2003). Enhancing victim empathy for sex offenders. *Journal of Child Sexual Abuse, 12*(3–4), 255–276. https://doi.org/10.1300/J070v12n03_10

Coetzee, L. (2020). Victim empathy in young sex offenders in the emergent adulthood development phase. *Journal of Sexual Aggression, 26*(2), 251–262. https://doi.org/10.1080/13552600.2019.1618931

Department of Youth Services (DYS). (n.d.). *Juvenile crime victim services.* Mass. Gov. https://www.mass.gov/service-details/juvenile-crime-victim-services

Foster, S. (2011). *Choreographing empathy: Kinesthesia in performance.* Routledge.

Gallese, V. (2009). Mirror neurons, embodied simulation, and the neural basis of social identification. *Psychoanalytic Dialogues, 19*(5), 519–536. https://doi.org/10.1080/10481880903231910

Hunnikin, L. M., Wells, A. E., Ash, D. P., & van Goozen, S. H. M. (2020). The nature and extent of emotion recognition and empathy impairments in children showing disruptive behaviour referred into a crime prevention programme. *European Child and Adolescent Psychiatry, 29*(3), 363–371. https://doi.org/10.1007/s00787-019-01358-w

Keysers, C., Kaas, J., & Gazzola, V. (2010). Somatosensation in social perception. *Nature Reviews: Neuroscience, 11*(6), 417–428. https://doi.org/10.1038/nrn2833

Leventhal, M. (2012, November 22–25). Moving towards meaning: The journey from creating in dance to a healing paradigm of dance movement therapy. *Proceedings from International Dance Council, CID: World Congress on Dance Research: The Dance Therapy Congress* Athens, Greece. http://www.marciableventhal.com/#!articles-and-publications/cqdg

Malti, T., Ongley, S. F., Dys, S. P., & Colasante, T. (2012, Winter). Adolescents' emotions and reasoning in contexts of moral conflict and social exclusion. *New Directions for Youth Development, 136*, 27–40. https://doi.org/10.1002/yd.20036

Montoya, R. M., Kershaw, C., & Prosser, J. L. (2018). A meta-analytic investigation of the relation between interpersonal attraction and enacted behavior. *Psychological Bulletin, 144*(7), 673–709. https://doi.org/10.1037/bul0000148

Office for Victims of Crime. (2005). The History of the crime victims' movement in the United States. https://www.ncjrs.gov/ovc_archives/ncvrw/2005/pg4c.html

Panda, P., Garg, A., Lee, S., & Sehgal, A. R. (2021, November). Barriers to the access and utilization of healthcare for trafficked youth in the United States. *Child Abuse and Neglect, 121*, 1–9. https://doi.org/10.1016/j.chiabu.2021.105259

Pennick, N. (2022). *The spiritual power of masks: Doorways to realms unseen.* Destiny Books.

Potter, N. N. (2004). Can sex offenders learn victim empathy in prison? In *Putting peace into practice: Evaluating policy on local and global levels* (pp. 55–75). Brill. https://doi.org/10.1163/9789004458772_009

Richardson, J. F. (2022). *Art as a language for autism: Building effective therapeutic relationships with children and adolescents.* Routledge.

Rizzolatti, G., Fadiga, L., Fogassi, L., & Gallese, V. (2002). From mirror neurons to imitation: Facts and speculations. In A. N. Meltzoff & W. Prinz (Eds.), *The imitative mind: Development, evolution, and brain bases* (pp. 247–266). Cambridge University Press.

Scholes, R. (Prods). (1994). *Once were warriors* [Motion picture]. Communicado Productions.

Sheets-Johnstone, M. (2010). Kinesthetic experience: Understanding movement inside and out. *Body, Movement and Dance in Psychotherapy, 5*(2), 111–127. https://doi.org/10.1080/17432979.2010.496221

Smith, A. (2017). *Facilitating victim empathy in counseling male sexual offenders: A strength-focused approach* (pp. 136–150). Routledge.

Stern, J. A., Costello, M. A., Kansky, J., Fowler, C., Loeb, E. L., & Allen, J. P. (2021). Here for you: Attachment and the growth of empathic support for friends in adolescence. *Child Development, 92*(2), e1326–e1341. https://doi.org/10.1111/cdev.13630

Trivedi-Bateman, N., & Crook, E. L. (2022). The optimal application of empathy interventions to reduce antisocial behaviour and crime: A review of the literature. *Psychology, Crime and Law, 28*(8), 796–819. https://doi.org/10.1080/1068316X.2021.1962870

Part III

Wearing a Mask

Chapter 10

Metaphors in the Mask
A Process of Exploring Personal and Professional Identities

Craig Balfany

Symbolic and Metaphoric Elements of Mask Making – Process and Product

Masks have a rich history in many cultures and have been used for various purposes, ranging from religious ceremonies and theatrical performances to social commentary and disguises (Second Face Museum of Cultural Masks, n.d.). In early Greek theater, masks were used as a means of expression before the introduction of spoken lines, allowing performers to tap into the hidden psyche and convey abstract imagery from the subconscious. Similarly, the donning of ceremonial masks has been used to shift self-perception, camouflage identity, and embrace a higher spirit. Picasso recognized the transformative power of masks when he witnessed Dan masks at an exhibition in Paris. He realized that the Dan artists were using masks to express their confrontation and conquer their inner fears, opening visionary communication channels and revealing hidden inner layers for others to witness. Masks became a metaphor for the presence of a hidden consciousness (Hood, 2021). The role of masks in healing and therapeutic practices has existed throughout history and across cultures.

Masks have played a crucial role in understanding "what it means to be human" by permitting the imaginative experience of "what it is like" to be transformed into a different identity or affirmed of an existing one. Overall, masks have been powerful tools for expression, communication, and self-exploration across cultures and periods (Edison, 2005). A mask can convey a person's apperception related to the subjective experiences and values that influence how an individual perceives themselves, others, and the world. These formative experiences also guide the development of an individual's strengths. These elements are often communicated via symbols and metaphors included in a mask. These symbols and metaphors serve various purposes, such as spiritual connection, transformation, and communication. Thus, masks can be an effective tool for use in different therapeutic modalities.

DOI: 10.4324/9781003365648-14

In contemporary Western medicine, masks used in healthcare and other occupational contexts serve protective purposes. In mental health contexts utilizing play, drama, and art therapy, masks have been used as a tool for clients to symbolize and express different parts of themselves or to externalize feelings or negative thoughts. Alfred Adler discussed the importance of an individual's "creative power" that taps into their potentialities to stimulate movement toward overcoming obstacles (Ansbacher & Ansbacher, 1956, p. 177). This creative power can be manifested in the mask making process. Adler believed that an individual is the artist of their personality, and their creative works reflect themselves (Ansbacher & Ansbacher, 1956). The creative process and finished mask can convey the participant's self-perception, approaches to compensating or overcompensating for inadequacies, and how their emotions catalyze their actions. Thus, the mask can enhance insight and self-awareness in a therapeutic or educational context.

The mask and mask makers highlighted in this chapter are connected to the art therapy profession. Their images demonstrate their creative abilities in using various media symbolically and metaphorically. Their courageous reflective narratives capture how the mask making process and product convey how life experiences influenced self and world views and the evolution of their personal and professional identities.

Mask Making – Media and Materials

As early cultures began to craft masks, they utilized materials that were accessible. The earliest surviving masks discovered in the Middle East, dating back 9000 years, are made of stone or seashells. Historically, mask making materials include clay, wood, bone, feathers, fur, fibers, and plant materials. Through trading with, or colonization by, other cultures, masks began to integrate new materials that reflected these cultural influences.

Contemporary mask making has an expanded array of construction materials, including paper/cardboard, synthetic clays, plaster, fibers, foam, plastic, and metal/wire. These materials influence the construction techniques and should be considered when determining the appropriateness for the mask making context. Many techniques can be used for building a mask. This chapter will focus on using plaster gauze to build a mask from a face. Other building approaches, using more accessible and less messy materials, can include pre-made face forms or constructing armatures from newspaper, foil, cardboard, or tape. A helpful resource on these building techniques can be found in the book *Making Masks* by Melody Anderson (2022).

Decorating and embellishing the mask expands upon a mask maker's material and expressive options. The options are only limited by the availability and the creator's application choices. These may include drawing media, paint, paper, photos/collage media, fibers, feathers, hair, beads, wood, plastic, found objects, metal/wire, and natural materials. The mask's purpose may influence the material choices used in surface decoration. If the mask aims to symbolize a particular animal, deity, social status, or identity, specific colors, shapes, symbols, or materials may reinforce the symbolic connection to the mask.

Expressive Therapies Continuum

The expressive therapies continuum (ETC), described by Kagin and Lusebrink (1978), classifies interactions with art media to process information and form images. This information is categorized in a hierarchical chart from the simple kinesthetic/sensory level to a perceptual/affective level, then onto a more complex cognitive/symbolic level. The creative fourth level can occur at the individual level or as a demonstration of the integration of all the ETC levels (Hinz, 2009).

Kinesthetic/Sensory Level

The kinesthetic component can be activated during the building phase of mask making. Engaging in the repetitive kinesthetic actions of cutting, placing, forming, and carving provides the creator with information on bodily rhythms, modulating tension, and allows for nonverbal communication. The sensory component focuses on the internal and external sensations experienced while using mask making materials (Lusebrink, 1990). Visual, olfactory, and tactile sensory channels can be activated when constructing a mask with clay, plaster, or wood mediums. A mask molded directly on a face is a highly sensory experience that enhances auditory sensations. This highly tactile experience, especially in partnership, can create a soothing and relaxed state for the participant. Some participants may express feelings of anxiety or vulnerability with a direct face-molded mask. It is essential to inform all participants about the timing, safety protocols, and steps of the process and to have frequent verbal check-ins with the participant. Utilizing plastic molds or pre-formed masks is an excellent alternative to forming masks directly from a face.

Perceptual/Affective Level

The Perceptual component deals with the figurative aspects and formal elements of visual imagery. This level involves translating mental activity into representing inner and outer experiences (Hinz, 2009). Materials such as clay, plaster, and wood often used in mask making are utilized at the perceptual level, and these media can expressively evoke form. According to Hinz (2009), creating a structured form from these materials can be calming, allowing participants to internalize their sense of self. The participant also engages in the perceptual level after removing a face-formed mask. They encounter the physical experience of seeing a three-dimensional model of their face that they can view from new perspectives.

The affective component captures the emotions aroused in the participant through their interactions with art media (Kagin & Lusebrink, 1978). Often, a mask making directive given in an art therapy session is framed as an expression of externally conveyed and internally held feelings, as well as dynamically reflecting externally and internally perceived images of the self. Powerful affective states may emerge as a participant comes face to face with feelings and messages they want to reveal or hide from the viewer.

Cognitive/Symbolic Level

The cognitive component facilitates the therapeutic use of problem-solving using art media. The cognitive level also includes the ability to classify the properties of media and sequence events in time (Kagin & Lusebrink, 1978). The cognitive thought process of mask making is intentional, including a high degree of planning and decision-making in manipulating art materials. This component engages the mask maker in reflecting on the past while anticipating the future.

The symbolic component concerns intuition, self-concept formation, metaphoric representation, and the expression and resolution of symbols (Hinz, 2009). Symbols integrated into masks contain elements that emerge from the mask maker's kinesthetic, sensory, and affective realms. The symbolic content can expand self-awareness, convey defense mechanisms, and connect inner meanings to outer experiences.

Creative Level

The creative level encompasses the fusion of information during the creative process. It can facilitate the integration of all levels of the ETC but can occur on any level. It synthesizes the participant's inner experience and outer reality during mask making. The creative level facilitates inventive and resourceful interactions with media that can lead to creative self-actualizing experiences.

Approaches to Mask Making

Engaging in and constructing a mask can be simple or complex, depending on the context, participants, and available materials. The media dimensions of mask making materials can range from soft, malleable, and fluid materials such as plaster, clay, and paper to hard or semi-pliable, rigid, and resistive materials such as wood, stone, cardboard, or metal (Graves-Alcorn & Green, 2014).

Simple mask making techniques include using pre-formed papier-mâché or plastic mask forms. Paper plates or cardboard surfaces can also be an easy mask foundation to build. More complex, time-consuming approaches that involve multiple steps include building with papier-mâché, sculpting clay or stone, carving wood, or layering plaster-infused gauze in a mold or on a face.

Pre-formed masks, usually papier-mâché or plastic, allow for accessibility to the activity if there are limitations in time, space, or fine motor skills. Constructing a mask, whether on a mold or directly on a face, supplies an added kinesthetic/sensory experience. The technique of building the mask directly on the face allows for a cooperative and collaborative dynamic between participants and the therapist. The experience can evoke a sense of vulnerability, trust, and attunement to non-visual sensory experiences for the participant.

Using plaster-infused gauze to form a mask directly from a face is a multiple-step mask making process. Prepare the plaster gauze by cutting it into one-by-six-inch strips; cut smaller strips to work around the nostrils as needed. Set the strips alongside a bowl of warm water. The participant can sit or lie on a comfortable surface. Use an apron or blanket to protect their clothes. Hair can be covered with a bathing cap. Before applying the gauze material, dampen thin paper towels with warm water. Lay the damp paper towels over the face, leaving the nostrils open. Once the mask is removed, the paper can easily be pulled off the mask's interior. An alternative approach is to apply a thin layer of petroleum jelly to the surface of the skin, eyebrows, and hairline.

After the participant is prepared, dip one gauze strip into the water at a time. Begin applying the strips around the outer edges of the face and work inward. Cut smaller strips to work around the open nostrils. After completing the first layer, gently smooth the plaster gauze to form it to the contours of the face. Repeat this process with a minimum of three layers. While applying the layers, be sure to have frequent check-ins with the participant about their comfort and inform them about the status of the building process. After the third layer has been applied, the plaster will begin to harden. When the mask form feels solid, it may still be damp; carefully assist the participant in lifting it off their face starting with the chin and jaw area. The entire application and setting process typically takes about twenty minutes. Allow the mask to dry completely before decorating.

Enhancing the Mask

Decorating and embellishing the mask is a creative opportunity for the maker to explore and experiment with various applied materials. Using paint and drawing media enhances the ability to convey facial expressions or external and internal affective states. The decorative process can go beyond the application of paint or glaze. Cutting, carving, and building up the mask surfaces enhance the dimensionality of the mask (Anderson, 2022). Applying collage materials allows the layering of images that may overtly or covertly express emotions and concepts relevant to the mask creator. Embellishment with three-dimensional materials can symbolically connect to their experiences and personal/professional identities. The materials used in building and decorating a mask can give the creator an occasion to engage with media across the ETC.

Exploring Personal and Professional Identities

Mask making can be an insightful experience for clients, art therapy students, and professionals. It allows the participant to explore varied materials while facilitating a creative and reflective process rooted in their identities and their intersection with their personal and professional identities.

This mask making experiential was used in a foundational course for art therapy graduate students. This structured directive introduced the use of mask making in therapy. It was an opportunity for them to work collaboratively and independently to experience using various media, from fluid to resistive. The participants were guided in the plaster gauze mask-forming technique and given options for forming armatures to enhance features or make textural alterations. By completing the mask, participants could symbolize elements of their personal and professional identities.

Each participant reflected on their kinesthetic and sensory experiences after using various media. Students discussed their perceptual and affective responses to the building process and their finished mask. Reflective writing was used to describe their cognitive process of creating the mask. Group discussions engaged the participants in describing their use of symbols and metaphors as an expression of their identities. Prompting questions were provided to facilitate their reflective writing. As one student stated, "The mask would become a self-reflection and serve as a visual symbol and metaphor relating to our life or life journey …" (Figueroa, 2022, p. 2).

The phase of decorative embellishment of the mask began with a semi-structured prompt: "decorate the surface of the mask in any way with any materials or found objects." Upon finishing the surface, ponder what might be "behind the mask" and then decorate the interior surface. The participants were then encouraged to reflect on the finished mask product. The reflective process could be facilitated with interview-style questions to which the individual could respond. Examples of prompts or questions may include: Describe the decorating process. What is the name of the mask? What does it show others on the surface of the mask? How might others perceive this?

What might be hidden behind the mask? How might the mask serve as protection? How does the mask reflect personal or professional identity?

Each participant could choose the depth and details they wanted to explore and express in their mask making process. One participant (Figure 10.1) wanted to use the outer surface "…to reflect the culmination of negative events I have experienced since maturing into adulthood" (Figueroa, 2022, p. 2).

The visual response to this theme was a textured and glittery theater-styled mask capturing youthful and ambitious energy, contrasted with a dark and dusky color symbolizing traumas that drained away their life energy. Despite the intensity of the participants' experiences, the mask embellishment process and the materials used allowed them to integrate, balance, identify strengths, and accept what has happened. Thus, they found new meaning in the beauty of the mask and the courage to follow their passions.

The contrasting inside surface (Figure 10.2) is painted black with luminous gold eyes and a disc on the forehead, symbolizing the participant's

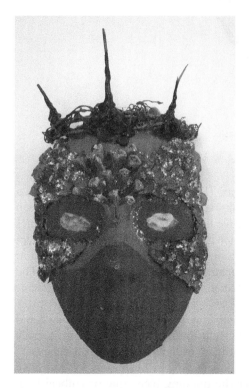

Figure 10.1 The front surface of Figueroa's mask.
Photographed by author.

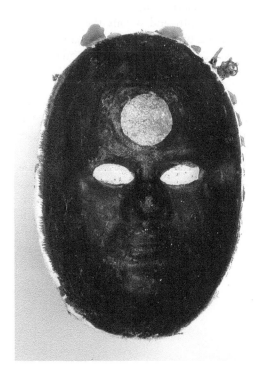

Figure 10.2 Inside surface of Figueroa's mask.
Photographed by author.

"love of the night time sky and moon" (Figueroa, 2022, p. 3). This internal darkness symbolically holds the mask maker in an ambivalent state between the love of the night and the reflective light of the moon, yet also becomes stuck in the shadows of darkness, which has become a comforting and protective place over time. This darkness contrasts with the experience of being in the "light," as it is associated with feelings of mistrust and vulnerability. The participant's reflective process created an opportunity to integrate and demonstrate self-awareness across the ETC's kinesthetic/sensory, perceptual/affective, cognitive/symbolic, and creative levels. Showing the mask and sharing the reflective narrative in a group setting was a courageous, socially interested act and a powerful and intimate experience for the participants.

Mask making can be a part of an ongoing self-care and self-reflective process for individuals. No matter the building technique or embellishing media used, masks can portray a current snapshot of what may be necessary for its creator to express or conceal from others. In Figure 10.3, the

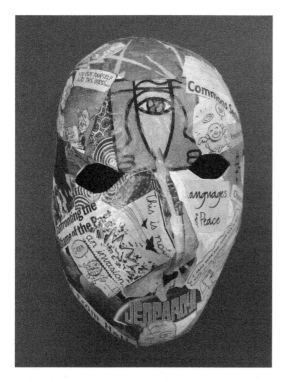

Figure 10.3 Collaged mask. Photographed by the author.

Photographed by author.

papier-mâché mask utilizes collaged images and words that are organized in a way that suggests a split face, with one side communicating messages of conflict, fear, shame, and consequences in contrast to the other side that conveys aspirations of love, hope, peace, sensibility, and finding a voice. This duality of messages captures the contrast between grappling with challenging experiences and emotions and the identification of the participant's strengths. This mask demonstrates and illuminates the navigation between work, relational, and social life tasks and their perceptions of self-identity and self-worth.

Conclusion

Mask making is rooted in the depths of human creative experiences that evolved from the need to understand, disguise, protect, express, and connect. It is a practical, experiential tool that can be used in the healing arts to elicit insight into relationships and self-awareness of personal and professional identities. The process and product tap into all levels of the expressive therapies continuum, allowing for creative opportunities to explore various materials and building techniques. Mask making encourages creativity and empowers expression, as every mask has a purpose and tells a unique story.

References

Anderson, M. (2022). *Making masks*. Melody Anderson.

Ansbacher, H., & Ansbacher, R. (Eds.). (1956). *The individual psychology of Alfred Adler: A systemic presentation in selections from his writings*. Basic Books, Inc.

Edison, G. (2005). *Masks and masking: Face of tradition and belief worldwide*. McFarland & Company, Inc.

Figueroa, R. (2022). *Experiential 4: Masks* [Unpublished manuscript]. Adler Graduate School.

Graves-Alcorn, S. L., & Green, E. J. (2014). The expressive arts therapy continuum: History and theory. In E. J. Green & A. A. Drewes (Eds.), *Integrating expressive arts and play therapy with children and adolescents* (pp. 1–16). Wiley & Sons.

Hinz, L. (2009). *Expressive therapies continuum: A framework for using art in therapy*. Routledge.

Hood, R. (2021, September 22). *Ceramics, sculptures, and visual art – From antiquity to contemporary*. Ceramics and Pottery Arts and Resources. https://www.Veniceclayartists.com/mask-the-art -of-concealment

Kagin, S. L., & Lusebrink, V. B. (1978). The expressive therapies continuum.*Art in Psychotherapy*, 5(4), 171–180. https://doi.org/10.1016/0090 -9092(78)90031-5

Lusebrink, V. B. (1990). *Imagery and visual expression in therapy*. Plenum Press.

Second Face Museum of Cultural Masks. (n.d.). *Masks in history*. Second Face. https://www.maskmuseum.org/masks-in-history

Chapter 11

Building Trust through Mask Making in East and West Jerusalem

Developing and Exposing, Disguising and Divulging Clinically and in Phototherapy Training

Tamar Reva Einstein

Yousuf Karsch (2003) compared the development of character with a photograph which is developed in darkness. In my 38 years in this world of expressive arts therapies, I can say that masks, either plaster or other kinds, are a powerful way to reflect and research identity, emotions, and transformation, whether in the training of therapists or clinical therapy. I have witnessed self-reflection, self-discovery, and trust building in ways that I believe could not be explored in the same intensity through other media. My clinical experience includes working on both sides of the city in West and East Jerusalem, Jewish and Arab. I found that the language and therapeutic use of art and artmaking provide a bridge between the complex and politically volatile line that invisibly separates the city. I was fortunate to work with diverse populations including Arab ex-prisoners, children of drug addicts, those in juvenile probation, and in training other therapists. In training other therapists and teachers, I was the Jewish female expressive therapist welcomed wholeheartedly into clinics, schools, and hospitals. No cultural masks were worn at all. This was a unique and rare, therapeutic, and human experience that will stay with me forever.

Different types of masks were used depending on a variety of conditions such as cultural restrictions, receptivity to appropriate touch, openness to experience, and depth of trust. For example, ready made white masks were chosen when working with those in juvenile probation, where touching was deemed inappropriate by staff. Court-ordered Arab youth engaged in mask making to help them contain expressions of anger and conflict, cultural beliefs, and confusion around identity. The masks created by the juvenile boys were often painted on the outside with symbols or colors of their ongoing, cultural, political conflictual lives, Palestinian flags, or the colors of the flags, while the inside was given less attention. For the adult ex-prisoners, I used plaster strips directly on their face. Their decorations included feathers, pom-poms, sparkles, and shiny paint as they engaged in play, and explored media and their joy alongside nightmarish childhood and adult memories.

DOI: 10.4324/9781003365648-15

Phototherapy and Mask Making

From the first camera obscura developed over 2,000 years ago, through analog and instant cameras, to the digital cameras used today, photography has been both an art form and a way to keep, collect, and document memories through visual images (Lefèvre, 2007). Phototherapy is the use of photography as a therapeutic tool in its many diverse forms (Shevchenko, 2015). For example, one might take photographs, have photographs taken, use found photographed images, family albums, and a mixture of all of the above (Weiser, 2004).

Masks share an even more ancient history than photographs; they have been and continue to be used in rituals, celebrations, holidays, rites of passage, and spiritual and religious healing ceremonies for thousands of years. Here, in Jerusalem, where the mask making and phototherapy course took place, there is a mask housed in a museum that is said to be 9,000 years old (Hershman, 2014). Both mask making and photography are integral parts of a wide range of self-reflective, expressive arts-based semester-long courses. Like the double exposures of analog photos, the unintended overlaps bring welcome surprises that enrich the learning experience and inquiry into the many layers of masks humans possess unconsciously and consciously (Keats, 2003).

As a photo therapist and teacher, I am inspired by the connections between the process of darkroom photography and mask making. Both require ample time in darkness for the process to come to light; both invite a time-related exploration in which each step invites the participant not to rush, to pause, and move at a slower pace. Film can be underexposed, overexposed, "burnt"; plaster strip masks can collapse, break, and crack when removed quickly, or be heavily layered or difficult to remove when left on the face too long. There is no perfect way to make masks, to take photos of the process, or develop the images. Each outcome brings an invitation to look deeper into whatever emerges and I often hear the question asked about both photography and masks in class, "How did I come out?"

Transformation

The rationale for this directive is that the making of the mask, the photographing, and continuing to change, ornament, embellish, develop, and engage with the process and product can help to deepen self-reflection on inner and outer selves. Students are invited to immerse themselves in the process of developing and exposing, disguising and sharing feelings, and identifying their symbolic language, alone and with group witnessing and holding the space for others. According to Dunn-Snow and Joy-Smellie (2000), therapists in training can creatively touch upon hidden and exposed parts of themselves physically and symbolically through mask making. Both metaphorically and literally, the masks and the documentation of mask making through the lens allow stages of development to emerge and be honored. The focus is always on transformation; improvising and playing with ideas, having conversations with participants on the process and meaning of their mask, dialoguing with the mask itself, and reframing the transformation (how it looks and feels). Students can zoom in and out, focus and refocus, look inside themselves with a wide lens or a narrower one, and become aware of the time and rhythm of each part of this experiential learning.

The Process

Once a year, the now frayed black cotton, cable knit turtleneck sweater is taken out of the closet and donned. This 13-year-old ritual signifies mask making day for the first-year phototherapy students in Jerusalem. Ranging in age from their mid-20s to 60s, this diverse group explores the use of photography as therapy in a two- or three-year training program. The introduction course is designed to encourage these participants to engage in multi-modal arts tethered in photography as the foundation. The mask making class usually comes toward the middle of the semester when the participants and instructor have become acquainted enough to build trust and play space in which self-reflective creative inquiry can safely be invited. The well-worn sweater becomes speckled with white by the end of this special double class of four hours from the plaster strips in this transformative experience.

After arriving in the classroom, we all set up the space and I describe what will happen: the sequencing, the possible emotions that might arise, how each student will be part of a communal ritual in which everyone will be in different stages of development in the plaster, like the darkroom process. How I will, as the facilitator, in my special garment, be making the masks on each one of the 12 participants one after another. Once their faces are covered, they will be led slowly to a waiting area, and they will be kept company by a fellow student. Students are told that they will be given a chance to photograph while not seeing. Because students are photographers, they are overly reliant on the use of sight, so this is an opportunity for them to explore other senses while taking a photograph without using their eyes. They will not be able to speak as the plaster warms up and dries, so all students are asked to be as quiet as possible so they become extra sensitive to signals given by the masked ones, especially if they become distressed by the process of their face being covered in plaster. Students are required to create a shared safe space and, as always in phototherapy courses, many photos will be taken by everyone present.

Applying and Removing

Plaster strips of different sizes, widths, and lengths are cut and stacked by size on the worktable next to tubs of very warm water. The tub is refilled as needed during the process of mask making. I invite all the students to cover their faces with petroleum jelly. This protective layer ensures that the masks come off comfortably. Students are already transforming visually. Hair is held back in bandanas and scarves, glasses are removed and clothes covered. A chair awaits the first volunteer, and we begin. Cameras are already clicking, the familiar sound of capturing a memory.

The plaster strips are dipped in warm water and gently pressed between my fingers to expel excess liquid. I place the first piece on the student's face with a firm yet delicate pressing motion (Figure 11.1).

This is repeated many times, leaving mouth and nose openings for last. I regularly check in with students along the way to ensure that they are comfortable, pausing, stopping, or continuing as directed by the student. Some students choose to have only one layer over the eyes to see a bit, some want to be completely in the dark, and have everything covered in three full layers. Once the mask is completed, students are led to the waiting area to rest while their mask dries. I begin another mask and slowly the room fills with people in different stages of the process. After 15 minutes, I begin removing the first mask. The cameras are out and ready. The removal is done gently; I slowly make sure to grasp the edges and allow the mask to fall away as I hold it. I hand the mask to the student to meet their plaster self (Figure 11.2).

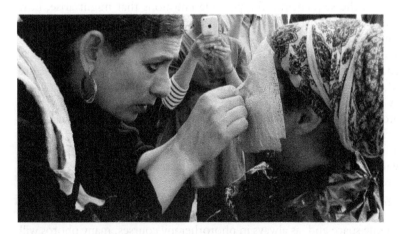

Figure 11.1 Applying plaster strips – cameras clicking.

Photographed by Magi.

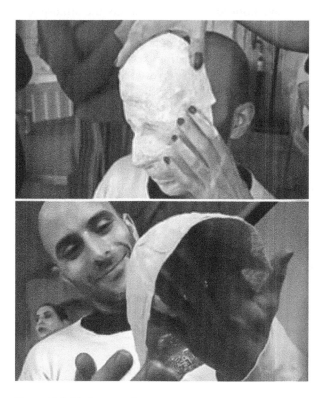

Figure 11.2 Mask removal.
Photographed by Rivka Rivlin.

There is often a quiet response, sometimes tears, laughter, amazement, or shock at the sudden light. In mask making, waiting, accompanying, witnessing, photographing, and finally writing are all parts of the process. Maggie, a graduate phototherapy student, reflected on her mask by writing:

"During the time of the building of the mask on the face the feeling was that everything slowly, slowly became screened, shielded, separated, outside life is blurred, and I move inwards to my most narrow, limited space.

Until everything goes dark, and there is no choice but to look inside, and to stay there in that inner place.

After some withdrawn minutes... the peeling begins.

An experience of renewal.

Of rebirth."

When the 12 students have all had their masks made and removed, the white plaster faces are lined up to dry with support on the windowsill or table. All the students write quietly and then we clean the classroom space and take a brief break. I have noticed that no one wants the atmosphere to change quickly or to venture outside the room for too long during this time. We then have a discussion and share thoughts about the process, the writings, photograph, and stories and associations related to their mask in a preliminary group processing. The group serves as a container for the sharing and all mask makers/photographers are the witnesses (Melson & Thurman, 1982). The students are told that the masks will go home with them for three weeks to be documented, transformed inside and outside with whatever materials feel right, and in whatever photographic manner they choose. An emphasis is put on the inner self and outer self, on how they want to amplify represent themselves and their mask. The masks are collected and gently placed in padded containers to take home, more photos are taken, and more associations arise. The students leave and I spend a moment in my plaster-decorated black clothes looking at the room, now empty of the students and their masks, another transformation. I reflect upon my first meeting with mask making in my own expressive arts therapy training in the 1980s, and I feel the lineage and continuity of the mask-making process (Figure 11.3). I remember the mask made at the completion of my doctoral studies and how important the process and product were in that rite of passage. I go home and shake off the plaster, but not the experience. The sweater carries all the years of each group even after the plaster is removed.

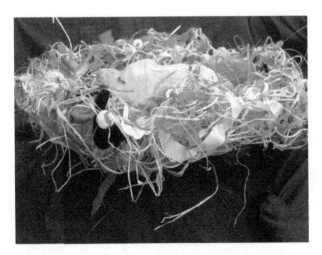

Figure 11.3 Me in my doctoral nest: Hands, heart, and head.

Photographed by author.

The Masks Return

The day the masks return is exciting, emotional, and visually daunting. I cannot list all the transformations here but can give some examples of how the masks returned. The photographs and videos of the processes were as astounding and moving as the physical masks. Masks filled with earth and seedlings growing, masks covered in rose petals that slowly rotted and dried, masks smashed to pieces and reconnected, bread baked in a mask over and over, or attached to a full plaster torso. Masks connected to another face on the other side, written in and on, collaged with photos, buried in dirt, and excavated, set out to sea, placed in a bowl of water and slowly disintegrated, not touched at all but moved around and photographed in different places, and with additions of glasses, makeup, openings, closures. Stories are told of trauma, rebirth, pain, beauty, becoming one's mother, regressing, growing, taking chances, trusting, fear, loneliness, freedom, expression, identity, loss, joy, and, in general, the transformative power the mask making summoned.

Afterthoughts

The phototherapy mask making and the masks returning are powerful individual and group experiences. In final papers, students deepen their understanding of what they learned in the process of making and witnessing. The community that was created in the class transforms relationships with each other and within themselves. When the pandemic began, it was obvious that such a class would need to end, but no one knew for how long. As of now, in 2023, it has not resumed. In all honesty, I can say that it is the class that I miss deeply and that has left me forever changed and transformed, as many students have reported in the years that followed. The slowing down that the ritualistic experience allowed, the intimate yet clearly delineated rules of physicality, the incredible work the students did through the lens of their cameras, and the lens of their souls is still with me. My fraying sweater has not been worn since 2019. It might become an artifact, carrying the memories and images that are forever developing in the dark room of the chambers of my heart.

In my clinical work in East Jerusalem, mask making has been an extraordinary experience on many levels. Many thought me mad or crazy to be working there, let alone touching people's faces while mask making. Perhaps Kahlil Gibran (2001) said it the best in the *Madman* when he felt blessed that his masks were stolen from him, and he was able to show his true self for the first time.

Unmasked and authentic, I was able to reach populations through mask making and the expressive arts therapies that would otherwise have been unreachable to me. For this, I am forever grateful.

References

Dunn-Snow, P., & Joy-Smellie, S. (2000). Teaching art therapy techniques: Mask-making, a case in point. *Art Therapy: Journal of the American Art Therapy Association*, *17*(2), 125–131. https://doi.org/10.1080/07421656.2000.10129512

Gibran, K. (2001). *The madman: His parables and poems*. Dover Publications.

Hershman, D. (2014, March–September). Face to face: The oldest masks in the world. The Israel Museum Jerusalem, 5–9. https://www.academia.edu/10230340/Face_to_Face_The_Oldest_Masks_in_the_World

Karsch, Y. (2003). *A biography of images*. MFA Publications.

Keats, P. A. (2003). Constructing masks of the self in therapy. *Constructivism in the Human Sciences*, *8*(1), 105. https://www.invaluable.com/blog/how-to-develop-film/

Lefèvre, W. (2007). *Inside the camera obscura: Optics and art under the spell of the projected image*. Max Planck Institute for the History of Science. https://www.mpiwg-berlin.mpg.de/Preprints/P333.PDF

Melson, S. J., & Thurman, W. (1982). The making of masks in psychotherapy. *Psychiatric Annals*, *12*(12), 1086–1089. https://doi.org/10.3928/0048-5713-19821201-12

Shevchenko, O. (2015). The mirror with a memory: Placing photography in memory studies. In A. L. Tota & T. Hagen (Eds.), *Routledge international handbook of memory studies* (pp. 294–309). Routledge.

Weiser, J. (2004). Phototherapy techniques in counselling and therapy--Using ordinary snapshots and photo-interactions to help clients heal their lives. *Canadian Art Therapy Association Journal*, *17*(2), 23–53. https://doi.org/10.1080/08322473.2004.11432263

Chapter 12

Encountering the Mask with Undergraduate Expressive Therapies Students

Engaging Ritual, Dialogue, and Reflection

Krystal L. Demaine

Like three threads of a braid, creative arts therapies (or expressive therapies) are grounded in the elements of play, creativity, and imagination; all of which are woven together lay a foundation and interconnection between art forms and practices within the field (Demaine, 2017). With the exception of music therapy, the other creative arts therapies require a graduate degree and training in a specific modality (art, dance/movement, drama, play, intermodal, etc.). Undergraduate degrees can offer a grounding in pre-professional practice, and a deepening of creative expression, expansion of self-awareness, development of interpersonal relationship skills, and formation of ego identity (Demaine et al., 2015). Students attracted to the study and practice of the arts in healing at the undergraduate level are often unique, creative, vulnerable, and intrinsically compassionate individuals. Quite commonly though, many of these students have developed an interest in studying how the arts heal because they or someone close to them has been healed by the arts (Demaine, 2017).

Experiential practice is intrinsic to learning about creative arts therapies, which involves an immersion into the therapeutic and expressive processes. Allen (1995) noted how there is a natural inclination to look inward and explore internalized experiences in (creative) art therapy. Through classroom experiences, students have a chance to examine inner struggles and the origins of such tensions. One of the essential ingredients in the development of self is the ability to be authentic and to engage in a place of truth; something that can be challenging to cultivate among young students but important to instill within the profession. Brené Brown (2015) said that "vulnerability is the core, the heart, the center, of meaningful human experiences" (p. 12). Arthur Robbins (1994) noted that in creative arts therapies, "it is rare that our unconscious does not spill out…" and that "accepting such vulnerability can offer a curative experience" (p. 145). While vulnerability may play a role in the classroom, it is also important in the clinical experience. After all, the classroom is an essential learning space for the developing therapist to best understand a client's perspective.

DOI: 10.4324/9781003365648-16

This chapter explores my experience teaching therapeutic mask making with undergraduate students majoring in expressive arts therapy (intermodal arts-focused). In discussing the students' involvement in working with the mask, themes emerge in the areas of identity and dialoguing vulnerability, image dialoguing, and invoking the unconscious, and permission to encounter. This chapter also reviews the application of masks using plaster cloth and other arts-based modalities, including letter writing and personal reflection, to engage in the meaning-making process.

Cultivating the Studio

Mask making as a teaching tool can serve a twofold purpose for the students. First, to educate in mindful therapeutic facilitation, and second, to explore the personal impact of the inner and outer representation of self. The mask making experience begins by cultivating a space for accessibility, community, activity, and inclusion within the studio classroom. The setting of the space helps to get the creative juices flowing. I prepare the space by hanging images of masks printed from the computer onto the studio walls. Mask making materials (sheets of plaster cloth, scissors, shallow containers of warm water, petroleum jelly, mask templates, hair ties or bandanas, cloth towels, and rolls of paper towels) are laid out on my large mandala tapestry in the middle of the room – a circle symbol that serves as a metaphor for the group as a container and space for witnessing and holding each other. I use this colorful mandala tapestry each year – one that my students come to know as the mask making tapestry. Students are asked to bring a yoga mat or chair and place it around the supplies on the tapestry in the middle of the circle.

I start the circle by telling the story of my early experiences with masks and mask making. Sharing stories is another way of cultivating space and modeling an authentic shared community. The story I tell begins when I was about eight years old, a time when I collected hand-painted masks. I acquired about 20 expressively painted porcelain masks of varying sizes and shapes and another set of papier-mâché masks which were decorated in fabrics and sequins. I hung these masks on my bedroom wall when I was young. Now, they are bundled and wrapped in newsprint and sitting in a box in my basement. I once adored those masks, fascinated by the intricacy and gracefulness of their design. I tell my students that as I grew older the masks that were in my life began to look different and took on a new role for me. When I was working as a music therapy supervisor at Mass General Hospital in 2004, I wore a medical mask to play music with my patients; and when my son developed a breathing condition in his infancy, I infused his albuterol through a plastic mask that I held to his tiny face every two hours for an entire year.

After I share my mask stories, I invite students to share and listen to each other's stories about mask making and mask wearing; they rekindle experiences from Halloween and masquerade parties to spa experiences involving exotic materials applied to the face for skin enhancement. After sharing some stories, laughing, and musing a bit, I read poems from Rupi Kaur, Khalil Gibran, and Shel Silverstein to set the intention of both the playful nature of the mask and the seriousness of the therapeutic intent. Then, I begin to show and explain the supplies that have been laid in the middle of the circle. I inform the group that we will be working with plaster material on their faces. For students who do not want to put both petroleum jelly and plaster on their face, I provide plastic templates for the plaster to be applied directly onto the surface. It is important for each student to learn about the material, how to instruct, apply, and understand what the materials feel like in their own experience. As long as no one in the class is allergic to plaster, we proceed as planned. I remind the group that there is a role for every person to participate in the mask making process.

The Masking

As the group settles into the space, music is chosen to set the vibe, something that the whole class agrees upon, offering an invitation to smile, be social, and dance if they wish. As people move around the room, bringing energy and organization to the space, I ask a few students to prepare shallow containers of warm water while others cut the plaster sheets into small pieces, some pieces narrow enough to fit on the tiniest areas of the face. I ask other students to take photos while the action happens.

The class size is usually between 10 to 15 students, just enough people so that each person can make a plaster mask during the two-hour studio time. I ask for one student to volunteer to go first, while the rest of the group serves as witnesses to the demonstration. The volunteer chooses where they would like to sit or lie while being masked; I suggest finding a place and position that will be comfortable for 20–30 minutes. In a workshop style, I explain the importance of preparation; tying loose hair back, covering clothing with a towel, and having extra towels nearby to catch dripping plaster and water. Students bring plaster pieces and warm water close to the demonstration space. I remind the volunteer student that their face will be touched to apply the petroleum jelly. Students witness the process of asking another to meet their space – in particular, the face can have specific vulnerabilities that require special permission to encounter. Particularly in a post-COVID-19 pandemic era and being conditioned to cover and protect the face from others, consideration for permission to touch another face is essential.

Once the student is ready, I apply a generous layer of petroleum jelly to the surface of the face and only to the areas where the student elects to have the plaster mask. Some students choose to create a mask that covers the entire face including the mouth and eyes, some choose a half-face mask, while others cover the top or bottom portion of the face only. The application of jelly is extremely important because applying plaster to the face without a jelly barrier would result in plaster sticking to the skin and a potentially harmful rash. I demonstrate by dipping a single piece of plaster sheet into the water and then applying it to the jellied face, smoothing it down, and repeating the process. The whole time I maintain a conversation with the student volunteer to ensure their comfort level while the class witnesses the process. If the water becomes cold, students in the class can refresh it with warm water; if water drips down their face, other students sop it up. Once the demonstration goes smoothly with the first student, others begin to partner up, and there is a steady current of activity in the room taking place until everyone has made a plaster mask. The mask takes about ten to 15 minutes to dry on the face and is lifted from the bottom up, with both hands on the cheeks of the face. After the mask is removed from the face or the plastic template, it is set aside to dry for a few more hours, as seen in Figure 12.1.

The Imaginal Dialogue

After the creation of the mask, it is time for the next level of transformation to begin. Students are asked to take the mask outside of the room, bring it

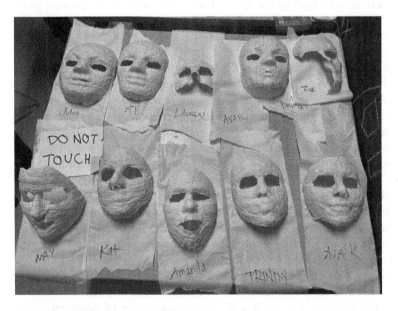

Figure 12.1 Plaster masks drying.

Photograph by the author.

somewhere for two whole weeks, and return it transformed somehow. Some students bring the mask to a completely unrecognizable state; cut into pieces or embedded within other materials. Others maintain the same form and decorate it with objects, paints, or other expressive materials. When the students come to the circle with their masks, I ask everyone to place the mask in front of them, along with their journals and writing materials. We start our engagement with the mask on a sensory level. I ask everyone first to look at the mask, then pick it up and feel it, hold it, smell it, and listen to it. Write down observational words, phrases, and images that offer a literal representation of the mask, of its texture, color, shape, or form. Next, I ask the group to begin to listen more deeply, as if the mask has something to say. Here is where an imaginal dialogue begins. I instruct the group through imaginal dialoguing to allow the mask to provide information, such as its name and gender, where it is from, where it has traveled to, its family of origin, favorite color, favorite movie, deepest fears, anxieties, pleasures, and hopes for the future. Write it all down. Allen (1995) wrote that the relationship with our imagination is a relationship with our deepest self; and that "working with the image process reveals that life is a series of multiple, overlapping realities, quite distinct from one another while also intertwining" (p. 108). Along similar lines, McNiff (1992) said that "outside the realm of psychosis, image dialogues deepen the creative process" (p. 109) and that "the artist realizes that the process of expression is never finished. It is an unending dialogue" (p. 105). As the students take this time to write, there is an emergence of a relationship, the inner and outer relationships of the liminal space between the self and the mask. The imaginal dialogue process is a method of narrative inquiry that evokes unconscious materials, eventually deepening into a relationship of knowing (Fang, 2020).

Meeting the Mask

One by one, the students introduce their masks, like introducing a friend to the class; giving each person a chance to meet the mask. One student holds up her mask and begins, "This is Eugenia. She is a 12-year-old girl from New England, and she lives with her mother, father, brother, and two dogs. Her life is happy but lonely and she is drawn to making art, drawing, and playing in nature…" Another student begins, "This mask has no name, they are shy and tend to hide in the shadows, that is why they are painted in dark colors…" The students are active witnesses and listeners when meeting these masks and practicing presence is key. Another student only shares a few remarks and timidly holds up the mask, reserving secrets that may be kept within. Other students are more boisterous, describing grand stories of a playful nature. While the sharing of the mask may be a true reflection of the self, the vulnerability of sharing what is within may stay reserved for another time. As McNiff (1998) suggested, many fear letting their emotions show through their work because they are concerned they may be perceived in a negative light. However, when students share narratives of a playful nature, they may tend to draw upon the creative spark within and the desire to engage in the imagination.

While the imagery of some masks may be literal in nature, others hold only private information. One student cut her mask into terse shapes and then reassembled them into an abstract form stitched together with red-colored yarn. Another student, whom I knew was working with a therapist due to trauma at home, ground down her mask into dust and bits, put the bits in a mason jar filled with red water, covered the bits with stones, and sealed the jar. She said, "This is Mask, they have no gender, and no identity, and they are crushed and covered by an indescribable weight..." Allen (1995) wrote that destruction is a necessary part of the creative cycle and that, while embracing the process can bring up fears, it can allow us to tap into the authentic place for discovery. McNiff (1992) says it is important to practice (expressive) art therapy without planning it out, to just allow for the emergence of things. And that "so much of art involves moving materials that already exist into new relationships with one another" (p. 143).

In a more literal sense, another student collaged words cut from magazines to the exterior of the mask. This mask, illustrated (Figure 12.2) below was named "Journey." The student told the group that Journey was "exploring her life authentically ... contemplation of faith ... perfection and future."

Once each student finishes introducing their mask, everyone, including the mask designer, writes a handwritten letter to that mask. The mask in turn receives letters from everyone in the circle. The letters reveal the reflection of truth and compassion for the life of the mask. My letter to Journey includes the following:

Dear Journey,

You have clear intentions marked by your words. It appears that your path is set out, but new paths may meander through, bringing new thoughts, inspirations, and words of intention. Where there may be narrow streams, you may stumble upon wide rivers to pass, this is all part of your process in the journey that it means to be you – this is part of your experience. You are preparing yourself for what is to come, for the unexpected, by grounding yourself with all possibilities. You are trusting yourself with this space and anticipating the unknown, the creative sparks, the improvised play, and the journey that is yet to unfold.

In gratitude,

Professor Demaine

Therapeutic letter writing can offer a rhythm of the truth between internal dialogue and imaginal dialogue, as there is a meeting of minds in the place between the imaginal and the subconscious internal. In the end, each student's mask receives several letters, one from every witness (student) in

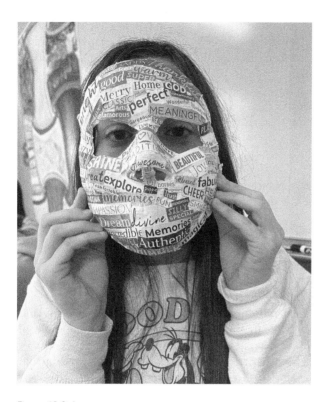

Figure 12.2 Journey.
Photograph by the author.

the group. Once everyone has shared their mask, and all letters have been written, the students take a few moments in silence to read the letters and to write or reflect in some way in their journals. I then ask each student to take a few more minutes to write a haiku in reflection of the mask making experience from start to finish.

Reflecting on the Mask

Before closing, I first remind the students of our collective experiences with the masks; rekindling how each mask shared a story, had an identity, and engaged in an imaginal dialogue. Each mask held a representation of self, a spark of creative freedom, and a palette for creative expression. Each mask brought a sense of authenticity, vulnerability, and a forum for teaching and learning. Finally, I note that the process of mask making invites responsibility, attention, care, and inclusion of others. Therapeutic mask making is a group process that relies on real group collaboration.

The mask making process closes with the students each sharing their reflective haiku poems. After the students take turns sharing their haikus as a final exaltation of their process, I share a collective poem, with phrases parsed from what I heard from each mask. The following shares my reflection on the group's haikus.

Wrapped in solid cloth
Cared, loved, holding space for you
Open, free, present

Touching my soul
Transformed without a sound
My fingertips graze the delicate fabric

Containing my memories
A space all parts of the self
Held with care, compassion, and warmth
You are heard.

The poem offers my final reflection and conclusion on the process and expresses my bearing witness to the container of the space and value of each group member. Mask making can be a serious practice and can offer an undercurrent of clinical experiences and the emergence of self-knowing. Mask making allows the students to explore the inner and outer and curate the identity-making that is palpable in the undergraduate expressive therapy studio.

References

Allen, P. (1995). *Art as a way of knowing*. Shambhala.

Brown, B. (2015). *Daring greatly: How the courage to be vulnerable transforms the way we live, love, parent, and lead*. Avery.

Demaine, K. (2017 January). *Teaching from a place of compassion in creative arts therapy* [Paper presentation]. Latin American Music Therapy Symposium. Panama City, Panama.

Demaine, K., Morrison, A., & Cardillo, N. J. (2015, October). *Undergraduate expressive arts therapy pedagogy: Cultivating culture and developing mindsets* [Paper presentation]. International Expressive Arts Therapy Association Conference, Hong Kong, Hong Kong.

Fang, N. (2020). Imaginal dialogue as a method of narrative inquiry. *Narrative Inquiry, 30*(1), 41–58. https://doi.org/10.1075/ni.18045.fan

McNiff, S. (1992). *Art as medicine: Creating a therapy of the imagination*. Shambhala.

McNiff, S. (1998). *Trust the process: An artist's guide to letting go*. Shambhala.

Robbins, A. (1994). *A multimodal approach to creative art therapy*. Jessica Kingsley Publishers.

Chapter 13

Working with Masks in Narradrama

Pam Dunne, Kamran Afary, and Ksenia Ilinskaya

Masks play a significant role as projective and distancing devices in drama therapy, offering a platform for therapeutic exploration. In his influential work, Landy (1993, p. 54) asserts that masks possess diverse forms and act as projections of the self. He describes masks as dynamic personas with sight and hearing, representing the individual in therapy rather than projecting characters. Landy highlights their transformative power, setting them apart from their conventional role in Greek theater.

Masks serve as tools for embodying various aspects of the self, fostering emotional distance and clarity, and providing a tangible representation of internal and external conflicts. They bridge the gap between the inner and outer worlds, enabling individuals to connect with their emotions, delve into the complexities of their identities, and promote personal growth and healing. Whether employed in drama therapy or psychodrama, masks offer a transformative medium for self-expression, integration, and self-discovery.

Narrative Practice and Narradrama

White (2007) applied Mikhail Bakhtin's notion that individuals adopt different social personas or roles to navigate various social contexts, which allows for a multifaceted expression of the self in the field of psychotherapy. He saw humans as living in continuous dialogue and constructing their identities through relationships with others, even when that moment exists only in their thoughts. Narrative practice focuses on the stories we tell ourselves, viewing the process as a movement from constructing a self-identity through a problem-saturated story to a multistoried world. White (2007) emphasized intentionality through identifying alternative stories that came to be known as preferred stories. Preferred stories, particularly when enacted with masks, provide a dynamic exploration of life narratives that diverge from the problem story. Within narrative practices, problem stories undergo transformation, leading to alternative stories that embody preferred identities. Mask exercises serve as a platform for silenced and culturally suppressed

DOI: 10.4324/9781003365648-17

identities to express themselves more strongly and become more visible (Hadley, 2013). Therefore, masks encompass not only concealment but also recreation and transformation (Magalhães & Martins, 2023). The special process of externalization invites the person to take a step away from the single life story. It is not the person who is the problem anymore, but the relationship one has with the problem. Masks help expand and deepen the externalization process to expose problems and their effects. They create more space between the person and their identity and story. Masks invite the participant to visually witness their expression of a preferred or unsilenced identity as well as to experience that preferred identity through concretizing their experience with embodiment in a way that is meaningful.

New preferred identities may become the basis for further development of the life story. This shift of exploring alternative stories/identities is more representative of peoples' intentions for their lives. Preferred identities convey the sense that we make a choice for something rather than for the problem. These preferred stories and identities "fit" with what people want for their lives and what matters to them.

Narrative therapy draws on theories and understandings by Vygotsky (1986), who recognized movements from the known and familiar territory of the problem to an area not yet known, but possible to know, of preferred stories and identities. Creating a mask of the known and familiar often leads to more understanding of the unfamiliar, and thereby reveals itself through questions that are asked of the known and familiar mask. These masks create a bridge, leading to the possibility to move from the known and familiar into the territory of the not yet known, but possible to know. White (2007) presented ideas about the "absent but implicit" connected with his reading of Derrida. Derrida (1978) focused on how we make sense of things, about how we "read" texts, and how the meanings that we derive from texts depend on the distinctions we make between what is presented to us (privileged meaning) and what is "left out" (subjugated meaning).

Narradrama unveils marginalized identities through storytelling and role-playing, emphasizing strengths and aspirations. Mask work is integral, with techniques like the problem mask for externalization separating individuals from issues, aiding insights. Silenced and personal agency masks encourage vocalizing emotions and connecting with hopes and dreams. Archetypal and transformative masks, like healers or visionaries, offer space for exploration and creative solutions. Embodying and moving the mask facilitate emotional responses and access to wisdom.

Narradrama embodies an intersectional approach, building both self-efficacy and self-advocacy through an intersectional lens. Narradrama practitioners work collaboratively to identify obstacles and overcome systemic oppression and dominant problem-saturated narratives that focus on deficits and pathologies. These narratives silence and erase our stories, worth, and values (Dunne et al., 2021a, 2021b, 2022).

Case Studies: Exploring Identity Using Distancing with Masks

To understand more about the development of using the mask to explore identity, here are some examples of group work based on play, non-direct methods, and distancing through creating masks inspired by nature, archetypes, animals, symbols, and fantasy characters. These exercises were carried out in the United States and in Europe in weeklong drama therapy workshops.

Exploring Nature and Masks in Italy and Switzerland

In Italy, group members struggling with expressing their identities created masks inspired by nature. For example, a tree mask (Figure 13.1) symbolized the participant's strength, motivating him to transcend his circumstances and embrace important values and life directions. Wearing his tree

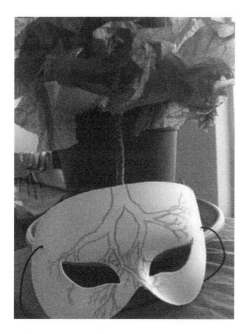

Figure 13.1 Tree Mask.
Photograph by Pam Dunne.

mask, he stood at the entrance of a door he had created, paused, and intentionally opened it, symbolizing the start of a new path.

Another participant combined a bird of paradise feather with colorful flowers in her mask, signifying focus, direction, and courage. This aspect of her hidden identity revealed a desire to be a pathfinder and courageous, which was often repressed. The colorful flowers surrounding the feather offered a diverse perspective, encouraging self-kindness. Through a musical image on her mask, she connected with her inner child's longing to play. Wearing the mask as her inner child, she playfully hopped on another participant's back and enjoyed being carried around the room in carefree abandon. Nature and play served as sources of inspiration for mask making, identity development, and the expression of preferred identities.

Nature both inspires and clarifies the role of masks. In Switzerland, participants displayed their chosen identity masks in natural settings and engaged in dialogues with them. Interviews with the masks were followed by a dance performance reflecting their inner essence. Participants captured images of their masks in the environment and held soliloquies. One participant placed her mask amidst bushes, near a rainbow, and alongside potted flowers (Figure 13.2). A photograph commemorated this moment, capturing the impact on the participant's life.

Exploring Myths, Masks, and Archetypes in Norway

In Norway, participants explored archetypes to better understand themselves and created molds of their faces which were used as imprints for multiple

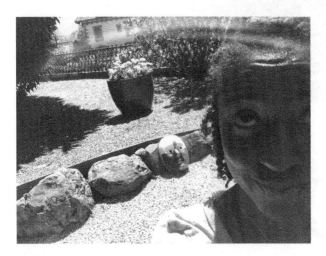

Figure 13.2 Mask in environment.

Photograph by Pam Dunne.

masks. Participants read myths, created their own myths, witnessed each other's stories, and reflected while moving as different archetypes. They created a specific environment with fabrics, objects, and art that suited the character of the archetype and began an exploration of that environment in the role. Each participant wrote and embodied their own myth, with other group members helping to integrate music, art, poetry, and color. One participant created a blue flowing fabric environment, like waves, which represented the calm and peace she desired. Her original archetype mask, Peacemaker (Figure 13.3), is a striking blue mask with stars surrounding it framed in an ocean of blue.

She made two additional archetypal masks: The Blue Goddess of the Sea, wearing a woven blue crown, with flowing, blue felt hair and golden eyes; and a Nurturer mask with water and leaf imagery. Placing the Nurturer mask on her face, the participant began to spontaneously move in an open, peaceful, yet grounded way, which was new for her, expressing to others that she felt safe and connected to her blue world and mask. She also explored the movement of the Goddess of the Sea, which invited a calm, deep movement related to breath work. A final collage highlighted a woven, wool

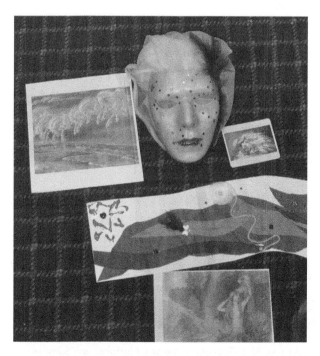

Figure 13.3 Peacemaker.

Photograph by Pam Dunne.

fabric base, ocean waves, and a threaded symbol made of yarn and fabric. Centered in this collage were the three archetypal masks in relationship to each other (Figure 13.4).

She referred to the culminating moment/collage as "the moment of happy surprise," and "mythical stories as waves becoming dolphins." Placing herself in the final image with the Nurturer mask, other group members created live sounds of the ocean and transformed into the waves. She discovered a new character, a butterfly, whispering to her (enacted by a group member): "let it go and be free; be sincere, reach, and be open."

US and Austrian Groups Explore Masks, Objects, and Creative Materials

In a workshop in the United States, a participant chose creative materials for mask making to represent preferred identities. She created a circular wire frame with a jeweled half-mask over her eyes, adorned with colorful flowers and feathers. The circular shape symbolized unity and flow, reflecting the deep emotions and desires that she conveyed through graceful, grounded, and confident movements. Still pictures were used to depict desired moments in her life.

In Austria, playful masks were crafted using balloons and various materials like fabric pieces, construction paper, felt, ribbons, and objects. Participants were prompted to explore longed-for identities and express them using

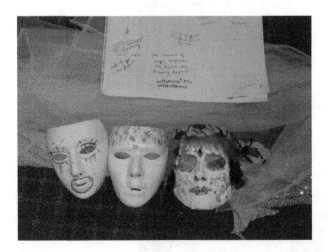

Figure 13.4 Archetypal masks trio: Blue Goddess of the Sea, Nurturer, and Surprise. Photograph by Pam Dunne.

creative materials. One participant surrounded herself with colorful balloons and fabrics, crafting a multicolored collage mask with balloon hair that she named "Reckless." Wearing a costume made of fabrics and ribbons, she danced freely in the balloon-filled environment, connecting with her suppressed longing for self-expression and recognizing its importance in her life.

Case Study Responding to Mass Incarceration in the US

This case study examines the use of mask exercises in a trauma-informed communication studies classroom at Lancaster Prison, where incarcerated men explored new identities of resilience to process social trauma and find hope in a maximum-security prison setting (Prison BA Initiative, 2018a, 2018b). The study aims to highlight the benefits of incorporating intersectionality in critical narrative interventions, guiding participants to expand their identities and reshape their self-narratives. Through mask exercises, incarcerated students developed facilitation skills to create new narratives and embody a more fluid sense of identity by externalizing stigmatized identities. The study included 25 participants, predominantly Black, Latino, and Asian men, along with White and Indigenous People, ranging in age from mid-20s to mid-60s, including first-generation immigrants and those serving long-term prison sentences, including life without parole.

The exercises focused on intersectional identities, addressing silenced or erased identities. Through masks, role play, and other artistic methods, students aimed to overcome societal stereotypes that portrayed them as disposable misfits and instead emphasized their critical communication skills as self-actualizing and accountable individuals working towards scholarly and professional goals. They staged a short play for incarcerated peers, faculty, invited guests, and family members, updating their self-narratives within their communities.

In the prison's bachelor of arts program, students used course materials to practice restorative justice and make amends. They initiated by embracing "externalization," rejecting the notion of fixed qualities and avoiding character correction. Course materials and research projects included performance and autoethnographic methods, strengthening their commitment to shift from punitive to restorative and transformative justice. By reshaping their life narratives and sharing scholarly works with wider audiences, incarcerated students rebranded themselves as California State University, Los Angeles bachelor of arts students.

As a prison educator, the challenge was to integrate ideas from the movement for the abolition of mass incarceration (Alexander, 2020) and punitive carceral regimes into drama therapy exercises (Davis, 2005). Students were encouraged to express their perspectives on the social construction of institutions and identities, including race, gender, sexuality, class, age, ethnicity, and religion. This work was informed by intersectionality essays (Crenshaw, 2007, 2016), a paradigm that recognizes how complex identities can be silenced or erased due to intersecting systems of inequality (e.g., racism and gender discrimination, heterosexism and ageism, class discrimination and ableism, etc.).

Narradrama mask exercises exploring intersectionality involved writing prompts and reflections on identity erasure, followed by mask creation to explore embodied images of the erasure and transformation experience. Masks were then utilized for narrative-questioning interview sessions, where students developed skills to facilitate dialogues using narrative questions as a key learning objective of the narradrama practice. Narrative questions counter the influence of dominant norms that pathologize individual qualities, emphasizing the social construction of shaping relationships. The masks were created during classes on various communication-related topics, such as interpersonal communication, health communication, performance and social change, and communication and social movements. Throughout role-play sessions with narrative questions, students embodied characteristics of resilience associated with the masks (Figure 13.5).

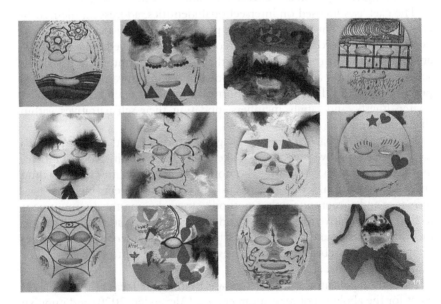

Figure 13.5 Masks of Resilience.

Photograph by Kamran Afary.

- Fostering a positive outlook on challenges as learning opportunities.
- Developing emotional self-regulation for appropriate expression of feelings.
- Prioritizing changeable aspects over uncontrollable ones.
- Identifying and reframing cognitive distortions.
- Cultivating qualities like humor to alleviate stress in oppressive environments.

They enacted roles using, for example, a three-part exercise inspired by Boal's (2019) *Theatre of the Oppressed*. First, they recreated a scene from an actual experience, then envisioned an ideal way they would have liked it to be, and finally, created a scene that mapped a transition from the actual to preferred moments. In doing these exercises, they took into account an ecological model of development (APA, 2017). Some of the questions they addressed to the masks included: What cultural institutions and social policies shape your interactions? How can you identify, challenge, or resist different forms of power, privilege, and oppression you encounter even as you are located inside a carceral setting? In one exercise, students used a modified version of the "six-part story making" (Lahad & Dent-Brown, 2012) of a hero's journey. For example, they created a plotline that expressed the student's resolve to strengthen their voice and to clarify their values and beliefs. These were shared with and performed in class. Some of the stories were then submitted by the students for publication to various peer-reviewed communication studies publications. Through their diligence and creativity, these incarcerated students help us pay attention to areas that need addressing, including advocacy, diversity, microaggressions, and resilience. Afary and Malone-Alteet (2022) and Afary (2020) provide examples of expressive exercises that explore the intersectionality of both a process and a goal.

Conclusion

Creating masks is crucial to the formation of new preferred identities in therapeutic and educational settings. Mask exercises in therapeutic and educational settings can open up space for an environment of play that allows participants to more fully engage in reflexive experiences while benefiting from a safe distance provided by masks. This, in turn, can deepen the ability to project the qualities that they want to embody. Mask exercises help participants gain a voice and liberate silenced or erased identities. Properly theorized and mindfully processed in a trauma-informed community of practice, masks can greatly help empower participants to find the strength and the skills they need to overcome oppressive norms and negative self-conclusions while moving towards expanding more authentic preferred identities.

We want to become better advocates for honoring and voicing silenced stories and preferred identities. Developing this legacy through aesthetic and therapeutic performances allows participants to explore, share, and honor authentic stories from their lives.

References

Afary, K. (2020). A Narradrama approach to teaching communication. In K. Afary & A. M. Fritz (Eds.), *Communication research on expressive arts and narrative as forms of healing: More than words* (pp. 3–31). Lexington Books.

Afary, K., & Malone-Alteet, E. (2022). Narradrama, intersectionality and devised therapeutic theatre in the prison communication studies classroom. *Drama Therapy Review*, *8*(1), 23–44. https://doi.org/10.1386/dtr_00091_1

Alexander, M. (2020). *The new Jim Crow: Mass incarceration in the age of colorblindness* (10th anniversary ed.). New Press.

American Psychological Association (APA). (2017). *Multicultural guidelines: An ecological approach to context, identity, and intersectionality.* http://www.apa.org/about/policy/multicultural-guidelines.pdf

Boal, A. (2019). *Theatre of the oppressed* (C. A. McBride, M.-O. L. McBride, & E. Fryer, Trans.). Pluto Press (Original work published 1974).

Crenshaw, K. W. (2007). Mapping the margins: Intersectionality, identity politics, and violence against women of color. In A. Bailey & C. Cuomo (Eds.), *The feminist philosophy reader* (pp. 279–308). McGraw-Hill.

Crenshaw, K. W. (2016, November 14). *The urgency of intersectionality* [Video]. TED Talk. https://www.youtube.com/watch?v=akOe5–UsQ2o

Davis, A. Y. (2005). *Abolition democracy: Beyond empire, prisons, and torture.* Seven Stories Press.

Derrida, J. (1978). *Writing and difference* (A. Bass, Trans.). University of Chicago Press (Original work published 1967).

Dunne, P., Afary, K., & Paulson, P. (2021a). Narradrama: A narrative approach to drama therapy. In D. R. Johnson & R. Emunah (Eds.), *Current approaches in drama therapy* (3rd ed., pp. 206–249). Charles C. Thomas Publisher.

Dunne, P., & Madrigal, R. D. (2021b). Narradrama as a three act play: Transformation, neurobiology, and discovery. *Arts therapies in international practice: Informed by neuroscience and research* (pp. 47–74). Routledge Books.

Dunne, P., Madrigal, R. D., & Afary, K. (2022). Narradrama as a three-act play. *Journal of Systemic Therapies*, *41*(4), 86–108. https://doi.org/10.1521/jsyt.2022.41.4.86

Hadley, S. (2013). Dominant narratives: Complicity and the need for vigilance in the creative arts therapies. *Arts in Psychotherapy*, *40*(4), 373–381. https://doi.org/10.1016/j.aip.2013.05.007

Lahad, M., & Dent-Brown, K. (2012). Six-piece story making revisited: The seven levels of assessment and the clinical assessment. In D. R. Johnson, S. Pendzik, & S. Snow (Eds.), *Assessment in drama therapy* (pp. 121–147). Charles C. Thomas Publisher.

Landy, R. J. (1993). *Persona and performance: The meaning of role in drama, therapy, and everyday life.* Jason Aronson.

Magalhães, L., & Martins, C. O. (2023). *Masks and human connections: Disruptive meanings and cultural challenges.* Palgrave/Macmillan.

Prison BA Initiative. (2018a, August 27). Imagine that [Video]. *Communication Studies Prison BA Journal.* https://www.prisonbajournal.org/copy-of-issues

Prison BA Initiative. (2018b, August 27). A fresh start [Video]. *Communication Studies Prison BA Journal.* https://www.prisonbajournal.org/copy-of-issues

Vygotsky, L. (1986). *Thought and language* (A. Kozulin, Trans.). MIT Press.

White, M. (2007). *Maps of narrative practice.* W. W. Norton and Company.

Chapter 14

Sexing the Mask

Explorations in Mask Making for Gender and Sexuality

Binyamin Rose

The face is an ever-changing site of expression, identification, age, ethnicity, gender, and sexuality (Fausto-Sterling, 2019; Lenoe, 2019; Rice, 2014). In its biological uniqueness, it has the power to define us, and can be adorned or altered to express our individuality or grouping (Klein, 2016; Valentova et al., 2017). In therapy with women and Queer people (people who do not identify with the heteronormative), I frequently hear comments about recognition and misrecognition, about the expectation to fit a particular gender model, of wanting to attract, or avoid attraction. Making masks has been a useful tool in my clinical practice to engage with gender and sexuality issues, from mask making with a young trans person who fantasizes about their looks, to the heterosexual cis-male as he explores the emotional world hidden behind the mask constrained by traditional masculinity. Exploring gender and sexuality in mask making reveals many complex layers in an interactive field of the personal and the interpersonal. This chapter will explore two experiences of mask making around the issues of sexuality and gender; the first account is about my facilitation of a group of professionals training to be Jungian analysts looking at clinical issues of identity. The second account is a personal arts-based research approach that explored my responses to the findings from the group and incorporated a more detailed mask making exploration of gender and sexuality.

My practice is informed by theory. Jung engaged with an inner world that contained layers of the psyche from the personal to the collective, from the conscious to the unconscious (Jung, 1931/1969). As Odde and Vestergaard (2021) reflect on this Jungian perspective: "[W]e may talk about the oneself, but the reality is that the self is a conglomerate of selves that are context-sensitive or context-dependent..." (p. 315). For Jung, this sharing in the collective by the individual experience reveals an inner world of archetypes whose images must be engaged and dialogued with (Jung, 1935/1966). From this standpoint, I began to engage with the notion that gender and sexuality are multi-faced, and that each layer contains important figures needing to be heard. Just as Jung in his renowned *The Red Book:*

DOI: 10.4324/9781003365648-18

Liber Novus (Jung & Shamdasani, 2009, p. 263) found a pathway into the depths which included gender play. I also found a need to work with a matrix-like constellation of masks to explore the role and meaning of gender and sexuality in my therapeutic work.

The Group Process

When I was asked to facilitate a short intensive course on gender and sexuality for a European group training to become Jungian analysts, the use of the mask seemed a natural choice. Mask making was chosen to help the students engage in a physical way in a weekend of theory and discussion. Developing from a brilliantly simple yet profound idea of Silverberg and Smyth's (2015) *Sex Is a Funny Word*, I asked the participants to use paper masks to draw two images, on the outer part of the mask, how they and others see their external gendered/sexual self in the face, and on the inside of the mask, how they view their internal experience of gender and sexual/ity.

A main idea of the mask making workshop was also to also provoke students to think and feel how their genders and sexualities are expressed and encountered in the therapy space. As can be seen in Gifney and Watson et al. (2017), Schaverien et al. (2006), and Young-Eisendrath (2004), the issues of gender and sexuality play a central role in the therapeutic relationship.

Prior to the session, the participants had a morning of talks and discussion on gender and sexuality from a theoretical perspective. Upon introducing the mask workshop, there was initially some confusion about what portraying their externalized gender and sexuality would mean. We engaged in a quiet and ambivalent discussion about the dynamics that sexuality and gender bear out in our faces. One participant said she felt deep discomfort in the initial stage – mask making was confronting something in how the world perceived her. Her gender as a sexed and sexual being felt frustrating, exposing, and forbidden. It also brought her to become more conscious of what she shows of herself to the world, and of what she hides in the expectation to be "more womanly." Indeed, a number of the participants felt that they had to tone down their experience of themselves. One participant said that he felt pressure to be reserved, not stand out, and to have a persona of being conservative and traditionally masculine, equating it with looking intelligent, trustworthy, and professional.

The group then turned the masks over and were requested to depict their inner experiences of themselves as gendered and sexual beings. From more "factual" self-portraiture (see Figure 14.1) on the outer surface of the masks, the trainee analysts began a wild and playful rebellion: the constraints were off, and the trainees made energetic animal markings, brilliant colors, psychedelic swirls, natural and supernatural images of trees, and cosmic third eyes. The mood in the room lifted and became more talkative,

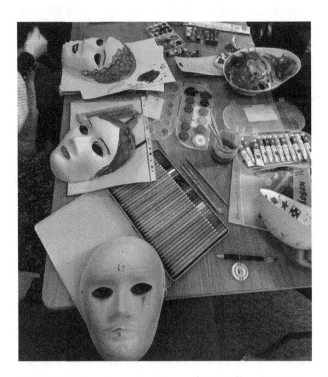

Figure 14.1 The group process on externalized gender and sexual identities.
Photograph by the author.

vibrant. A male candidate painted big red inner lips, and a forehead full of color. His mask, like a few other participants, began to use paint which flowed outside of the inner mask and began to show on the outer (Figure 14.1). He described a sense of release and yet of fear about showing this to the outside world. One participant began to confront how much was being contained and the possibility of containing less.

An experience of frustration and failure evolved in the messiness of constructing the mask. Some of the participants complained that they couldn't get the right image or the right colors, the paint shot out, or the color was not strong enough. The loss of control, the failure to perfect seemed to resonate with the recognition that our inner images often fail in the desire to curate a particular stable image of the Self. It brought a recognition that, just as others might fail to identify our gendered and sexual selves, so too do our self-perceptions, or rather desires to look a particular way or attract, fail. It felt like the process had begun, a mourning, a letting go of our inner images of ourselves (Figure 14.2).

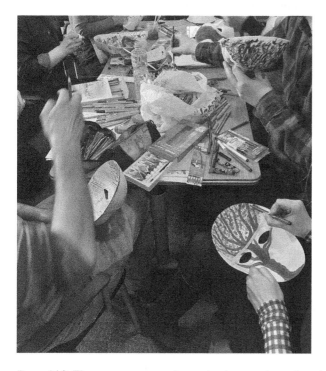

Figure 14.2 The group process on inner visual expressions of gender and sexual identities.
Photograph by author.

In the conversation after the mask making, the participants began to ask important questions both as human beings (what does my gender and sexuality mean?) and as nascent Jungian analysts (what does it mean to be a gendered and sexual being in a deep therapeutic relationship?). The discussion seemed to show a development of deeper empathy with the people they worked with, as they could feel their own disorientation towards being seen as gendered and sexual. The opening up of this dialogue between maker and mask effected an important conversation afterwards. Questions after the mask making revolved around emotions of containment, exposure, of recognizing the problem of attempting to be a blank screen, whilst also asking how much space one's gender and sexuality takes up in the therapeutic relationship. The classic image of the poker-faced analyst began to disintegrate in favor of a deepening awareness that the face is ever-shifting, ever communicating. Curiosity stirred about what the mask provided as a third space of personal and collective reflection, a place of mutual creating which mirrored the way gender and sexuality are constructed.

Taking the Process Further Through Arts-Based Research

The group had given me much material to process. I decided, encouraged by McNiff's (1998) text, *Art-Based Research*, to put myself into a personal process. I wanted to see, after years of practicing and working with Jungian theory in Queer spaces, what would emerge from a detailed, first-person experience of gender/sexuality mask making. One area that constrained the group mask making workshop was the use of a single mask. Jung's (1935/1966) notion that sexuality is nascent, polyvalent, and germinal, ever-developing, rarely static, and many-faced, confirmed my sense that sexuality and gender have distinct yet interlinking roles that need to be clarified. I was limited in what I could bring to a workshop in another country. What would I do if I had more time and resources? I saw potential for an interactive mandala of masks, masks that allowed room for different expressions in different situations. Beyond the binary of inner and outer, I found that different masks could be used in different interactions. Reflecting on the process, a list emerged in my journal:

- The outer mask constructed by others
- The outer mask(s) I portray to others
  - the sexual
  - the gendered
  - the roles of professional, parent, friend, citizen...

The masks of physical experience – kissed lips, dilated pupils of the eyes, blush
The inner masks of gender – the subtle body, intermediate, in-between images
The inner masks of sexuality – the zones of pleasure/desire
The wished-for face which I didn't get – the idol on which the real is sacrificed
The most interior, the mask of my soul – does the soul have a body/sexuality/gender?

My initial conflict was around what this multiple-mask making series might do. Would it endanger the fluidity of the actual psyche/soma, trying to pin down an image causing it to concretize? Would it limit the experience of sexuality and gender by categorizing the different layers? Alternatively, could the masks become more momentary, photo-like documentations, portraying snapshots of the soul and body? A space to engage and recognize an emotional psycho-somatic experience of one's gender and sexuality in the ever-shifting encounter through time.

Moving from the conceptual to the material, I identified a need for a variety of art supplies – from delicate tissues and transparent silks to raw materials such as clay, wool, metal, mirrors, and slime. I also needed prefabricated images, photos, porn, and erotic texts for collage, as well as materials for writing and painting. The different materials, in my fantasying, created a parallel with the genetic materiality of the body, which served as the bedrock of the mask base-frame and the secondary layering stages of what was done with or on top of it. The prefabricated images and words served as a further layer or aspect of introjecting, which allows the mask maker to engage and acknowledge the influence of the world around them.

Two Masks

As I prepared the room for mask making, a sense of anticipatory anxiety began. Avoidance and fear: could I really be doing this? And then, a recognition of the mundane objects became pregnant with potential meaning. From the process, two masks stood out as having significance, although I can well imagine that others would find different masks as profoundly expressing aspects of the person's sexual and gendered Self.

Mask of the Outer Body

Using clay to express the outer mask of physical appearance that others see was striking. The clay seemed to resemble qualities of the skin, the smoothness, the unwanted bumps and lumps, a sensual experience of the surface of the skin and flesh. The molding brought to the fore the changing nature of the contours of the face. A desire arose to create something "attractive" to conform and to remold. Already, I became aware of how the fantasy, the social, and the physical quickly entwined; reality was a negotiation.

Once finished, I found myself wanting to wear the mask whilst wet. Profoundly, I felt this dead weight laid on top of my face, its cold and damp materiality aroused both a sense of mortality and revulsion. The mask also created a blindness, an experience of being forced behind a veil, a space to encounter the in-betweenness and provoke questions of ownership (Figure 14.3). If the layer of the mask is a me-not-me experience, then behind the veil could emerge a potential space, confined but still potential.

The making of the mask did not cease once it had been constructed. Poetically, the drying process created significant cracks. There was a sense of triumph in the cracks appearing: the breaks and ruptures allowed space for other things to slip out, that an expansive sense of the body could be given

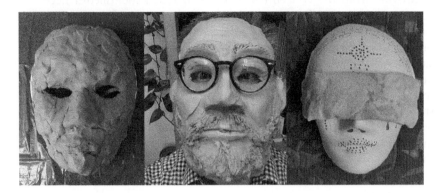

Figure 14.3 The personal process from the beginning of external gender on the left, to the external mask of inner sexuality on the right.

Photograph by author.

room. It also provided a letting-go of the static sense as the mask dried, changing beyond the control of the human hand. A worry that it would totally crumble emerged in me, a nevertheless persistent drive to preserve the physical form. It made me sit with the tension of loss of self and moving beyond the limits.

The Inner Sexual Mask

Despite Freud's making conscious of the sexual taboo and the swinging 60s, direct expression of sexuality is still challenging in the therapy room. The pathologization or resistance to calling kink an addiction or a perversion belies the diverse sexual practices and their experience on the couch. The use of metaphor or words often helps to ease the person into such intimate details of pleasure and desire. Discussing kink, fetish, and graphic acts of sex can produce shame and avoidance even the experienced therapist and patient (Elliott, 2020; Schaverien et al., 2006). The vulnerability of making the sexuality mask was immediate. Even in the privacy of my own space, alone, I was confronted by the need to use the reverse side of the mask which would not be seen if worn. I wanted images, porn, objects of sex, zones of pleasure, and yet, working through the taboo was not so easy.

Each step required an inner permission: to print pornography, to engage in choosing images, to tackle a sense of respectability which stood at odds with the sensuality of porn, and to deal with its stickiness attaching itself to the meaning of glue and paint. The desire to create a collage, to weave two or three images together to obscure the images, brought an intense awareness of how, after over 25 years of working in the Queer community, engaging in the real experience of externalizing one's own sexuality can feel frightening and vulnerable when placed in a visible, interpersonal domain. I also wondered about the ethics of what it would be for a person I am working with to bring their own sexual images. Some masks are made and cannot be shown. Questions should be asked about why this is so in a Queer, sex-positive world, a working through of the concomitant shame – what does the person learn from the reluctant shame?

The inner section of the sexuality mask seemed, blushingly, complete, stuffed with external images and yet, where was the space for the zones of pleasure, the no-go zones, the zones of negotiating with the Other? My thoughts turned from the inverse of the mask to the front/seen mask. As others might find, working with sexual introspectiveness is balanced with a dialogue with what gets shared with another, and the external part of the mask became a very different experience. The external face of the mask became a blindfolded image, a hiding of the eyes, with markings and words. Making dots that soon emerged like tribal signs, yet warning signs, signs of recognition and signs that remained ambivalent. The markings fell on zones of the mouth, ears, and forehead. From the intense and passionate inner world came a much plainer, almost minimalist, image. The external spaciousness balancing out the interior seemed to mirror much of the experience of the group where trainee analysts found they filtered out a colorful and vibrant inner life to portray an outer mask of the normal, respectable, and traditional.

Discussion and Conclusion

The two processes described here are a testament to the flexibility of the act of mask making. Simple or complex, with limited or boundless resources, the mask making workshops have the capacity to dig deep into the visceral and unconscious experience of gender and sexuality with therapists with a range of professional experience. Mask making was a versatile therapeutic act of raising consciousness, providing a play space that challenged the maker to not just think but to feel and experience what it means to be a gendered and sexual being and how that plays out both internally, with self-awareness, and collectively, how the inner experience relates to the different relationships around. From the feedback from the group, ironically, the masks seemed infectious, a number of participants wanted to take the activity and do it with their partners, spouses, a friend, or their clients. Engaging therapists in the workshop helped them develop confidence to think more creatively about how they work in therapy around sexuality and gender. For the facilitated group, it also helped to challenge previously held notions of what a therapist is/does and provided a space to see the impact of gender and sexuality of the therapist in the therapeutic space.

Both the group and my personal mask making drew out some of the important questions of how and why identity is constructed. Bringing to image showed the impact of defenses used to protect the sexual and gendered selves. Likewise, the physicality of the mask making was a vehicle for making sexuality and gender not only expressible through metaphor but also through the felt sense and visceral experience. The masks helped bring to light the painful choices of hiding wonderful, colorful aspects of who we are, as well as allowing the pleasure of private intimacies to be seen and to invigorate the notion of what it is to be a sexual being.

Creating these images brought deep emotions to the fore, of shame, regret, desire, sensuality, and feeling sexy, and allowed room for fantasizing how the balance could be different. The masks, especially in the personal research, created a network of images that evoked a dialogue of how these different selves link together. The images worked as both confirmations and confrontations of the many-faced Self; to encounter parts that reside undervalued in the shadow, but which perhaps are key to the wholeness of being human. To recognize oneself as many selves also brings the possibility of letting go of fixed notions of what one needs to be, to allow a play space for other selves to come in. As can be seen in both experiences described, the masks highlighted how the communal world interacted heavily in constructing sexual and gender identities. The masks are witnesses to how much the person has been shaped by the social realm. Yet it reminded me of Jung's words about masks, that they can be given by the community to be worn by the individual, as a means to heal the collective (Jung, 1934/1966, p. 150), and that perhaps these masks heal by allowing the participant a gap between the collective and the individual to break through and create something anew.

References

Elliott, C. (2020). *Existential kink: Unmask your shadow and embrace your power.* Weiser Books.

Fausto-Sterling, A. (2019). Gender/sex, sexual orientation, and identity are in the body: How did they get there? *The Journal of Sex Research, 56*(4–5), 529–555. https://doi.org/10.1080/00224499.2019.1581883

Giffney, N., & Watson, E. (Eds.). (2017). *Clinical encounters in sexuality: Psychoanalytic practice.* Punctum Books.

Jung, C. G. (1931/1969). The structure of the psyche (R. F. C. Hull, Trans.). In H. Read (Series Ed.), *The collected works of C.G. Jung* (Vol. 8, pp. 139–234). Routledge and Kegan Paul.

Jung, C. G. (1934/1966). The relations between the ego and the unconscious (R. F. C. Hull, Trans.). In H. Read (Series Ed.), *The collected works of C.G. Jung* (Vol. 7, pp. 123–241). Princeton University Press.

Jung, C. G. (1935/1966). Principles of practical psychotherapy (R. F. C. Hull, Trans.). In H. Read (Series Ed.), *The collected works of C.G. Jung* (Vol. 16, pp. 3–20). Princeton University Press.

Jung, C. G., & Shamdasani, S. (Ed.). (2009). *The red book: Liber novus.* W.W. Norton and Company.

Klein, U. L. (2016). Eighteenth-century female cross-dressers and their beards. *Journal for Early Modern Cultural Studies, 16*(4), 119–143. https://doi.org/10.1353/jem.2016.0034

Lenoe, M. (2019). The semiotics of the face in digital dating: A research direction. *Digital Age and Semiotics and Communication, 2*, 17–40. https://doi.org/10.33919/dasc.19.2.2

McNiff, S. (1998). *Arts based research*. Jessica Kingsley Publishers.

Odde, D., & Vestergaard, A. (2021). A preliminary sketch of a Jungian socioanalysis – An emerging theory of combining analytical psychology, complexity theories, sociological theories, socio- and psycho- analysis, group analysis and affect theories. *The Journal of Analytical Psychology, 66*(2), 301–322. https://doi.org/10.1111/1468-5922.12667

Rice, C. (2014). *Becoming a woman: The embodied self in image culture*. University of Toronto Press.

Schaverien, J. (Ed.). (2006). *Gender, countertransference and the erotic transference*. Routledge.

Silverberg, C., & Smyth, F. (2015). *Sex is a funny word: A book about bodies, feelings and you*. Triangle Square.

Valentova, J. V., Varella, M. A. C., Bartova, K., Stebova, Z., & Dixson, B. J. W. (2017). Mate preferences and choices for facial and body hair in heterosexual women and homosexual men: Influence of sex, population, homogamy, and imprinting-like effect. *Evolution and Human Behavior, 38*(2), 241–248. https://doi.org/10.1016/j.evolhumbehav.2016.10.007

Young-Eisendrath, P. (2004). *Subject to change: Jung, gender and subjectivity in psychoanalysis*. Routledge.

Part IV

Healing the Wounds

Chapter 15

Super Art Therapy

Michael Boyce

My love of superheroes started when my mom introduced me to Wonder Woman on the television when I was four years old. I was enamored with this woman who, when sensing danger or trouble, would spin around and in a flash of light and thunder, twirl into this amazing character in a colorful costume. Her golden tiara, protective bracelets on her wrists that deflected bullets, and magic lasso on her hip that, when thrown around someone, compelled them to speak the truth. She was kind and strong and confident. Through Wonder Woman, I discovered the world of superheroes. I loved these larger-than-life super friends who went from adventure to adventure, fighting bad guys and trying to always do the right thing in these fabulous costumes, but they would also hide their unique and dazzling superhero personalities behind a mask of normalcy. I thought that if I was Wonder Woman, I would be Wonder Woman all the time!

Superhero Identity

The superhero concept created by Jerry Siegel and Joe Shuster was born in 1938 with Superman, who in his secret identity of Clark Kent wears a set of glasses and contorts his body to look smaller than he is. In this identity, Kal-El (birth name) portrays a fumbling klutz to mask the strength and power of his alien heritage as Superman. Wonder Woman similarly would hide her identity as an Amazon princess behind the "mousey" mask of Diana Prince, the ugly duckling secretary in a man's world. Bruce Wayne's cowled mask was that of a bat, a creature of the night. When he dresses as Batman, he strikes fear into criminals, righting the wrongs to avenge the murder of his parents who were murdered in front of him when he was 8 years old.

I discovered the Marvel superheroes as a teen, much different than the DC superhero world, with real-life issues. These heroes were created in the 1960s at a time of social upset and proud activism. They were interpreted as signs of the time, representing a variety of marginalized groups and individuals. The X-Men were mutants who "were born this way" and were hated

DOI: 10.4324/9781003365648-20

and feared by the world they were sworn to protect; they were rejected by society at large but they still tried to help everyone in their superhero tights, even the people who hated and feared them. Spider-Man was a nerd who struggled to make rent and had a sickly aunt and was picked on by the other kids in his secret identity as Peter Parker. The Thing was considered a monster because of his rocky appearance and people ran in fear of him. Superheroes were a sign of hope, always trying to keep going and doing the right thing even when the world seemed against them. Superheroes wear masks to disguise themselves and to protect them from the world that they fight for (Lee, 1962).

Duality of Identities and Masks

Superheroes have always represented dual identities, masks, and the hero's journey. I could relate to this duality of "wearing a mask" as a queer youth. At the age of eight years old, only my superhero identity was considered deviant and wrong. I am thankful that I had the medium of comic books and superheroes to help me make sense of something that was so heavy and complicated to my adolescent self. I was able to compartmentalize that I had a secret identity that I had to protect from a very dangerous world that made it very clear how they believed biology was supposed to work. For me, being able to relate my lived experience to the template of superheroes saved my life.

My origin story with art therapy started as a child when I used art and drawing superheroes as therapy. As a young queer child who grew up in a small Midwestern conservative town, I felt isolated and different from all the other kids. The world seemed scary and very against being different from the established social norms. Turning to superheroes and drawing was a therapeutic escape to a world where being different meant that you could be a hero and stand out in a proud and positive way. Comic books were a sign of hope, always trying to keep going, never giving up, and having a positive mindset that things will be OK in the end. Unbeknownst to me, I was practicing art therapy. I resonated with Wonder Woman through the lens of a stranger from a strange land, being different, standing out, the visual imagery, the symbolism, and my interpretation. Later in life, I recognized the queer iconology of the character. I have worked with many vulnerable populations, ages eight to 60 years old, who struggle with belonging and feeling the overwhelming experience of being rejected and marginalized by the world around them. It is particularly heartbreaking when a mother or father rejects you for being different because of your gender identity or sexuality. It is also incredibly hard for someone to feel the hatred in someone's eyes because of the color of their skin or how they are perceived.

Super Art Therapy

Mask wearing is embedded in our culture. It represents mystery and intrigue when connected to a masquerade party or festival and celebrated, and it can be protective and decisive, as in the recent global pandemic and hospitals. Masks are a part of ritual, ceremony, and performance. I quickly adapted my own version of art therapy, incorporating masks into my work with many different populations. I use mask making to connect with multiple populations and to explore and help with processing and help in redefining someone's place in the world. It can enable clients to see themselves versus the way they allow the world to see them. The exploration of identity in art therapy can help someone gain a deeper understanding of themself, as well as reinforce self-worth and build confidence.

My superhero art therapy origin story mutated when I went to art school in San Francisco. I created a comic book superhero origin story for my lived experience. This prompt was self-created as part of my major that combined illustration and graphic design. I found creating my origin story to be therapeutic in processing my childhood trauma and seeing the experience from a new perspective. Combining art and therapy was further explored when I created a children's book to explain the difficult subject of homelessness as my graduation thesis and gallery showing. Creating this book to help children understand that people who are unhoused are still people and to help take away the "other" component was very rewarding and well received, and my superhero helping identity was born.

Becoming an art therapist to help clients in their healing seemed like the perfect superhero persona for me to explore as a career. With this newfound power, I then went to graduate school for counseling and art therapy. For my thesis in graduate school, I explored the effects of art therapy on expressing one's identity among individuals who were unhoused and living at a shelter. I incorporated my super art idea into the thesis with a superhero illustration directive to explore identity. This was the cornerstone of my presentation. Creating a superhero identity was met with an enthusiastic response by all participants and really helped them to feel hopeful and positive about the future.

Superhero Directive

I have used super art therapy with individual clients, groups, and workshops with marginalized communities, people who feel they are the other, who don't feel they belong in our complicated world, such as people in the LGBTQ+ (lesbian, gay, bisexual, transgender, queer or questioning, intersex, asexual, and more) community. These sessions are always well received and popular as a safe space for communities that continue to struggle with rejection and exclusion. The superhero client, group, or workshop can explore identity and strength to find a new perspective, personal growth, and better understanding. Super art therapy is an avenue for healing and empowerment. It can help clients to identify their power and enhance the superhero that lives inside them.

The directive prompt is "What is your superpower? Give it some thought... what is your superpower?" That very loaded question is usually how I start a session with a new client. If a client struggles with this question or says they do not have a superpower, the magic of art therapy comes in and helps to unlock these barriers. I help many different populations by bearing witness and helping them to find their own strengths and superpowers.

Comic Book Narrative

The superhero comic book narrative approach starts with asking clients to create a childhood memory. If the client is a child, I will ask them to draw a moment in time from their memory that stands out to them. The client then draws the moment, and we process the drawing. We look for patterns or themes that emerge in their art. I ask the client how the art they created makes them feel, and what it felt like to create it. With the client, we analyze the meaning behind the art and how it relates to their current, past, and future selves. After bearing witness to this art making, which can take multiple sessions depending on the individual, I then prompt the client to take that memory and use it to empower them in the present moment by creating a super version of themselves. I then give them an additional prompt of "what is your superpower?" After processing what they want or feel is their superpower, I ask them to draw themselves as a superhero. Responses to this prompt depend on how far a client would like to explore and push themselves. I have had some clients create whole origin comic books for themselves, something I did at art school.

A Client's Story

While working at a dialysis center, I would meet clients who had to sit at a machine which filters their waste products from their blood so that they can live. It is a time-consuming and emotionally draining process, and my job as an art therapist was to engage with any of the clients who were interested in creating art while stuck in the chair for four to six hours, three times a week. Typically, the clients would opt out by saying they did not know how to draw or that they were not an artist. My response was to explain that the beauty of art therapy is that you do not have to be a trained artist or have any experience with art; all that is needed is imagination and a desire to create (Figure 15.1). Art therapy channels the childhood instinct to explore with a crayon and a piece of blank paper. I started working with Melvinda at the dialysis center, and one of my prompts was to draw a childhood

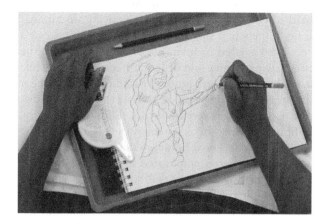

Figure 15.1 Pencil drawing of a female superhero.

Photograph by the author.

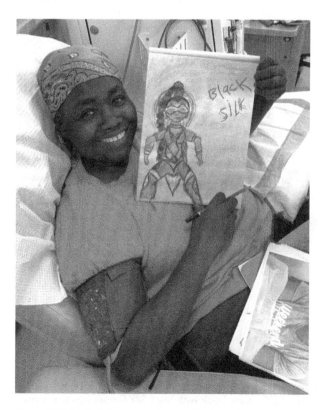

Figure 15.2 Melinda lying on a hospital bed and her artwork of her superhero, Black Silk.

Photograph by the author.

memory. I did not ask for a positive or negative memory and left it up to her. She drew herself at the age of four years old experiencing discrimination and racism for the first time when she wanted to buy a milkshake at a drug store counter. She was so excited to be in her favorite dress with the grown-up responsibility of having money and ordering herself a drink while her mom shopped. The white counter clerk ignored her, and Melvinda kept waving the five-dollar bill at her, but the clerk acted as if she did not exist. Melvinda teared up as she processed this very traumatic childhood memory, and she was surprised at how she remembered so many details, down to the yellow ribbon in her hair and the checkered linoleum flooring.

I helped Melvinda process this very complicated and hurtful memory using empathy, unconditional positive regard, and congruence. The next time I worked with her, I prompted her to create a superhero drawing to reclaim her power, and she loved the idea. Melvinda's eyes sparkled as she quickly came up with the costume and mask for her alter ego and she was so excited and proud of herself for her hard work (Figure 15.2). She came up with a character with a strong superhero name who had a karate chop and stood up to racism. This superhero drawing helped Melvinda to reclaim her narrative of feeling invalidated and showed her the strength she had within. Her superhero drawing was even the centerpiece to an art therapy art show as well as a video short about her experience (Figure 15.3).

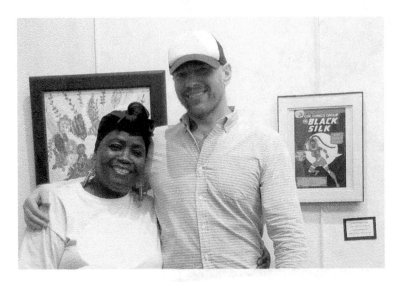

Figure 15.3 Melinda and Mike standing in front of an exhibition of artwork with a mockup copy of a CDC comic book with Black Silk featured on the cover.

Photograph by Stacey Hauser.

Conclusion

The superhero directive is a very simple concept of being your best self, or a magical-thinking version of who you would want to be. Most individuals are familiar with the superhero, certainly over the last few decades, with them dominating the public mind in entertainment media through film and television. The superhero directive, focusing on one's strengths instead of weaknesses, is an empowering approach to art therapy. Wonder Woman said, "We can't help the way we're born. We can't help what we are, only what life we choose to make for ourselves" (Bardugo, 2017, p. 102).

References

Bardugo, L. (2017). *Wonder woman: Warbringer 1*. Random House Children's Books.

Lee, S. (1962). *Amazing fantasy*. Marvel Comics.

Siegel, J. (1938). *Superman*. DC Comics.

Chapter 16

Painting Masks, Reflecting on Gaps

Student Veterans Explore Internal and External Realities During an Art Therapy Group

Maru Serricchio-Joiner and Einat S. Metzl

Many veterans who return from active duty deal with post-traumatic stress disorder (PTSD), traumatic brain injury (TBI), eating disorders, and other associated mental and physiological symptoms (Ferrell et al., 2021; Jones et al., 2018). PTSD and TBI within the military have been a focus of research; however, the focus on gender differences in the expression of trauma is minimal, especially as it impacts veterans integrating back into the civilian world. This integration has been found to evoke feelings of isolation, confusion, lack of trust, and a sense of identity disconnect (DeLucia, 2016). Hourani et al. (2014) looked at gender differences when expressing traumatic experiences during active duty, showing women expressed more distress and were more likely to experience and report PTSD symptoms, while men were more likely to be exposed to traumatic events than women. Further, men were found to externalize their trauma and show distress by engaging in substance abuse or self-harm. Veterans tend to need social and mental health support when returning from active duty; however, they are known to be hesitant to access support and resources such as therapy, veteran center services, and financial and academic advising (Albright et al., 2017; Oberweis & Bradford, 2017).

Meaning of Gender Within Military Culture

The relationship between gender and the military has rarely been researched, as the military has been traditionally seen as a male space (Egnell et al., 2019). While in the last decades the social construct has developed and transformed, females, femininity, and women's roles within the military continue to be a "perennial struggle" to integrate (Oppermann, 2019, p. 113). Women are increasingly being recognized as a crucial aspect of the construction of maintaining and fighting for peace and safety in the world, and with that recognition has come a push to understand the differences in gender perspectives (Egnell et al., 2019). Oppermann (2019) suggested that the gender perspective integration was still being understood and

DOI: 10.4324/9781003365648-21

implemented, and while women have been "disguised" as men within the military structure, they are seen as an auxiliary role to men. The differences in the expression of trauma within the military suggest a difference in vulnerability, as men reported more externalizing disorders such as substance abuse, irritability, and impulsiveness, while women expressed more numbing and avoidant symptoms (Hourani et al., 2014). These gender differences were seen within this group during the mask making directive and are discussed in more detail later in this chapter.

Group Art Therapy for Veterans

Group therapy has been highlighted throughout multiple publications as a supportive environment and service for veterans, as it provides a sense of safety and belonging that individual therapy may not offer (Jones et al., 2018; Smith, 2016). The expression of trauma through art making, and the physical nature of it, has been determined to assist in unlocking memories that are difficult to verbally share and easily integrate within one's identity (Campbell et al., 2016; Smith, 2016). Further, mask making in particular has a way to create, cover, hide, transform, or reveal identity expression (Dunn-Snow et al., 2000). Mask making is known to be a transformational experience and helpful through transitions and change.

The Group Setting

In 2020, an art therapy group was created and offered to students at the University of California, Riverside campus who self-identified as veterans. The group consisted of seven UCR students and one alum, all ranging from 18 to 40 years of age. The purpose of the group was to provide a safe space among veterans, to decrease isolation, and support integration into civilian life. During pre-interviews, participants all reported a desire to feel a sense of belonging and be seen. All participants committed to weekly two-hour sessions for group art therapy lasting for a total of eight weeks. No participants were excluded from the group, regardless of any prior diagnosis or other co-occurring conditions. This chapter focuses on the mask making directive and its process. Mask making was deliberately introduced during week four. It might be important to understand the responses (the art creation and later verbal processing) were also contextualized within the whole eight-week program (See Table 16.1). Specifically, during the third week, the week before mask making was introduced, participants delved into their trauma narratives for the first time. Participants stated that after sharing their trauma narratives, there was a release of emotional burden. Participants came back to Week 4 and felt lighter and much more connected to one another. This level of connection was much different than in prior

Table 16.1 An eight-week protocol group art therapy intervention for veterans

Art Therapy Group with Veterans	
Number/Type of Session	*Description*
Session 1: Group (120 minutes)	**Building rapport and goal setting** Discuss informed consent, sign forms, and fill out paperwork. Engage the group in psychoeducation, goal setting, and create a sense of safety. **Art:** Explore art materials and create an image/symbol that represents you and what you would like to get out of this group.
Session 2: Group (120 minutes)	**Transforming stress through receptive attention** (Martin, 2013) Mindfulness skills: Awareness of breath meditation with guided visualization (Martin, 2013) Psycho-education: Visualizing and referencing a personal image of a calm place in order to reduce stress reactivity (Martin, 2013) **Art Task:** Safe Place Collage (Campbell et al., 2016)
Session 3: Group (120 minutes)	**Visual trauma narrative** **Art:** Create six images Trauma Narrative: (five to seven minutes for each) 1. Last time before the trauma that you felt safe 2. The moment right before the trauma occurred 3. Trauma 4. Moment right after the trauma 5. Next time you felt safe and peaceful after the trauma 6. Representation of the last time you self-soothed (this can be abstract and/or symbolic)
Session 4	**Address and identify symptoms and triggers** (Campbell et al., 2016) **Art:** Mask Making (external and internal aspects of the self)
Session 5	**Dialogue** (Campbell et al., 2016) **Art:** Using images of self before trauma and image of self after trauma **Writing:** Create a dialogue between the two
Session 6	**Identify grief and loss caused by combat trauma, and opportunity or gain** (Campbell et al., 2016) **Art:** An image that represents the loss you experienced and the opportunity
Session 7	**Integration** **Art:** What are you taking from the group?
Session 8	**Closing** (Martin, 2013) **Psychoeducation:** Review of the program **Art Task:** Co-create "circles of mindfulness" drawings with shared drawings of appreciation for all participants. Mandala piece exchange, create one with all participants' pieces. **Closure:** Group discussion about the experience of the eight-week process

group sessions. Week 5 offered participants a way to deepen their understanding of what emerged in the mask making through writing and verbal processing. Thus, all participants engaged in writing a dialogue between the person they are today and the person they were before their military trauma exposure, while exploring the mask (inside-outside masks) they made the previous week.

Mask Making

All participants engaged actively, talking to each other while engaging in the art, and gravitated towards painting and mostly stayed with one medium (Figure 16.1). This was the first group session in which a participant was absent; however, it was also the first group session in which participants appeared less tense than usual. The participant who was absent, JS, made sure to create her mask the following week, to stay on track with the group. It was clear at this point in the group that participants had developed a rapport and the safety to be vulnerable with one another. As mentioned prior, this session directly followed the group session in which the trauma narrative was addressed. Participants reported they felt a sense of relief and lightness and entered the mask making with ease.

All participants chose their pseudonyms prior to beginning the group. A participant who chose to identify as Nodnarb for this research explained that he felt embarrassed that as a man in the military, his traumatic was not related to combat. Nodnarb compared himself to the other men in the group, and men in general within the military world, who truly had fought for their country. He unmasked himself throughout the art process by showing the internal softness, kindness, and array of bright colors he associates himself with. Nodnarb explained that his outer persona is dark,

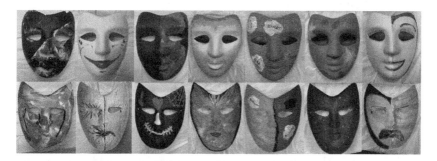

Figure 16.1 Masks (Nodnarb, JJ, TLG, Paige, JS, Eleven, Momma Bear).
Photograph by Maru Serricchio-Joiner.

camouflaged, within a military world where men are expected to show toxic masculinity as a form of strength. Nodnarb experienced closeness and relief in sharing his true self, discussing in the post-interview that he experienced the group as "collectively messy," going from being alone with the mess to a collective mess, to a place of connection and love.

Similar patterns emerged when participant TLG created a half-black and half-camouflaged outer mask as well as depicting the camouflage with military colors. TLG followed Nodbarb's expression of softness by stating that while he was in combat, he also felt he needed to only show his strength. Furthermore, TLG stated to the group that he was a loving person and even sometimes cried, as represented by the heart symbol and tears in the inner part of his mask. TLG expressed a deep need for forgiveness and attempts to make meaning of traumatic experience within the context of veteran life when engaged in written dialogue.

> You don't know it now, but you will never be the same. A part of you will be stuck in that time and place for the rest of your life. It is not necessarily a good or bad thing. There are elements of it that are both. The way you perceive the world and how you behave for the rest of your life will be indicative of this experience. That first slow, steady, squeeze will have irreversible effects. Permanent results. Nothing that used to matter matters. My desire for sex, money, and glory [is] replaced by a want of peace and forgiveness. My fear is replaced by understanding and that understanding will destroy everything you think is pure, innocent, beautiful. Your calling will emerge from all of this. A devotion to protect those who can't protect themselves. The evil you experienced will follow you every day for the rest of your life.

The women in the group had similar dichotomies; however, their external expression was "flowery, bright, sunny, and caring." Females discussed how their traumatic event was not related to war or fight-related events. Participant Eleven stood out in the group from the beginning phases, reporting that her military trauma was different from others. Initially, Eleven did not express much related to her experience of sexual abuse in the military and created images that clearly stated she felt alone, isolated, and unable to connect to the world. Eleven described her experience as a veteran student as one of panic and loneliness. She felt as though everyone that looked at her had no idea what she had experienced and wondered if they could really see through her initial persona. Eleven initially engaged in the group process in a very guarded manner, similar to what her art expressed. Eleven would engage in the artwork; however, at times she would not want to share with the group what she had created (Figure 16.2). However, during week four, there was a shift in Eleven's engagement. Week 4, mask-painting

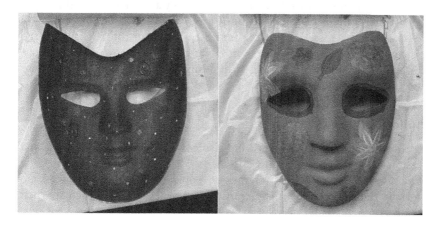

Figure 16.2 Eleven's mask making.
Photograph by Maru Serricchio-Joiner.

directive, was the week after the trauma narrative week. Eleven engaged and opened in a way she hadn't before. Further, the week after mask making, Eleven wrote a letter to herself.

> To me, you do not owe anyone an explanation. You are beautiful, but that is no one else's business. Stand strong and stand your ground. You are not here to be cute and innocent, to be adored and stared at. You have the right to tell someone off and you have the right to be angry. If it makes you uncomfortable, that is not okay and do not feel the need to justify a terrible situation. You can say no, you can leave, you can change your mind. Do not feel bad for upsetting someone else when they clearly never cared about how you felt in that situation. At the end of the day, it'll be you who suffers, not them... Do not protect someone simply because they are liked, or they are higher ranking. If it's wrong, it's wrong. There is no gray area... You are amazing and people who matter will see that. Learn to love yourself and stop relying on others to bring you happiness. You matter too. Love, Me

All in all, during this session a gender division appeared in both discussion and artwork, showing differences in what participants felt were expected to express externally versus internally. Participants who identified as male often utilized this art directive to describe external strength and hardiness, while internally, they verbalized their images as depicting hurt, anger, and at times sweetness and other "feelings that society might associate with weakness, such as silliness and love" (e.g., JJ's masks). At the same time, female participants seemed to depict a dichotomy as well, but one that man-ifested differently: expressing feelings of guilt, sadness, and complexity on the inside of the masks, while the images painted on the outside focused on beauty, nature, bright colors, etc. The dialogue focused on internal/ external communication as well as differing societal gender expectations and norms.

Implication for Practice

In reviewing the group dialogues and visual narratives around mask making (Session 4) and processing those (Session 5), three main themes may be relevant to the experiences of veterans on a university campus in general and can assist those working with veterans to further clarify and articulate their unique experiences and needs.

1. Seeing oneself in the mask of another: Mask making can reduce isola-tion, support meaningful socialization and belonging for veterans who are students.

The common bond, clearly found in prior studies as well (e.g., Jones et al., 2018), came across as participants discussed the decrease in isolation simply knowing that others in the group also suffered in some similar ways. The psychological isolation in which most participants resided was also noted by the team when observing participants' art, which did not include social engagements, family support, or friendships in their images, which is uncommon for university-age group participants. In fact, when they described their safe spaces, those were all places where they were alone, often in nature, and removed from "the threat of others." The need for connection but also the fear of deeply connecting with others, despite their blemishes, traumatic experiences, and needs, were expressed verbally and creatively through the mask making process. As previously found in litera-ture, art making promoted a sense of purpose and opportunity to express emotions usually internalized (DeLucia & Kennedy, 2021). For men and women who have experienced painful and hurtful experiences with others (through war, the military system, sexual abuse), it may make sense to focus on opposing needs to connect, heal, as well as defend or fight. The tension between such opposing needs creates a deep clinical conflict, which partici-pants could begin to explore through reflecting on their images of inner and outer realities, inner and outer masks, and the tensions/gaps within.

2. Looking inside and out: Masks can assist with identity formation and cultural adaptations in transitioning from the military system to the uni-versity campus.

A second theme that arose from reviewing the art, clinical notes, and the experience as a student veteran on campus was feeling unlike their fellow students culturally, feeling out of time or space, having been immersed in a vastly different system with norms focused on the shared rather than individual wellbeing, with firm rules and structure, and with a much more behavioral (and less emotional or creative) focus. These challenges were named as a main motivation in seeking support within the veterans' services on campus, and the shared sense of responsibility participants named for the wellbeing of others in the group, especially around making sure others who were struggling continued to attend. Participants also articulated a sense of identity loss or identity confusion, resulting in both negative (isolation, drinking) and positive (seeking therapy, choosing to engage in academic work, engaging in art making and sport) coping skills. Emerging from this theme is a need to clinically focus on developing an individual identity, where previous identity foreclosure or identity confusion is felt. In this way, the masks integrate the shared present self while also allowing participants to explore aspects of self which were linked to their veteran, student, and often unexamined psychological identity pieces, to enhance an authentic and integrated sense of self.

3. Gender differences in mask making (process and product) in our veteran group suggests the need for a gender-informed perspective and interventions.

An important theme arising from this exploration includes the often-differing experiences of men and women who serve in the military. While not always the case, most women serving in the military do not serve in direct combat operations (thus, are less likely to endure combat traumas), yet women soldiers are much more likely to endure sexual harassment and sexual abuse during their service compared to male soldiers. While there are clinical benefits of sharing differing experiences, at least for participants in this program which was brief, the differences seemed distracting and brought contradicting needs. Male participants stated that there was not enough shared experience of combat trauma to fully explore it and named that they felt out of place or unable to contribute to their fellow (women) participants who endured sexual traumas. Similarly, women participants were able to bond together and point to gender biases of the military system, but that often shifted the focus from the needs of combat veterans to feel appreciated and understood for their part in the operations. Specific barriers to empathy, emotional expression, or perceptions of possibilities in civilian and military engagements might also be heavily impacted by gender norms and roles.

As noted above, while all participants utilized the masks to explore differences between external and internal experiences, a gender difference emerged that is likely related to societal expectations: for male participants, the differences were between emotions that are perceived as more masculine on the outside, while internally they named feelings associated in society as feminine (sadness, vulnerability, etc.). For women, the outside of the masks often depicted concrete aspects of their physical identity as they believe they are perceived, while internally they recognized the multilayered emotional and relational aspects of themselves. In this way, masks allowed participants to explore how societal expectations shape how others perceive them, what they have internalized, resisted, and what aspects of themselves remain hidden/unknown to others.

Conclusion

In this research study, verbal and written responses, facilitated by mask making, explored belonging and identity formation in a civilian world that can feel isolating. While group art therapy can provide corrective experiences of inclusion and validation, this study found that there were gender differences when expressing military trauma, suggesting a need for gender-informed perspectives and interventions. Combat and military experiences have been seen through a gender binary lens for decades, disregarding the complexities of military narratives (Christensen, 2021). While in this study, mask making assisted with identity formation and cultural adaptations in transitioning from the military system to the university campus, further research would aid in understanding the intricacies of past military experience from a gender- and trauma-specific perspective. Continued research is also recommended in the powerful way art making, and mask making specifically, can help veterans in the task of separation-individuation as they integrate into civilian life.

References

Albright, D. L., Fletcher, K. L., Pelts, M. D., & Taliaferro, L. (2017). Use of college mental health services among student veterans. *Best Practices in Mental Health*, *13*(1), 66–80. https://www.researchgate.net/publication/319839482
Campbell, M., Decker, K. P., Kruk, K., & Deaver, S. P. (2016). Art therapy and cognitive processing therapy for combat-related PTSD: A randomized controlled trial. *Journal of the American Art Therapy: Association Art Therapy*, *33*(4), 169–177. https://doi.org/10.1080/07421656.2016.1226643
Christensen, W. M. (2021). Breaking the binaries in security studies: A gendered analysis of women in combat [Review]. *Contemporary Sociology*, *50*(3), 236–238. https://doi.org/10.1177/00943061211006085o
DeLucia, J. M. (2016). Art therapy services to support veterans' transition to civilian life: Thestudio and the gallery. *Journal of the American Art Therapy*

Association: Art Therapy, 33(1), 4 12. https://doi.org/10.1080/07421656.2016.1127113

DeLucia, J., & Kennedy, B. (2021). A veteran-focused art therapy program: Co-research to strengthen art therapy effectiveness. *International Journal of Art Therapy, 26*(1–2), 8–16. https://doi.org/10.1080/17454832.2021.1889007

Dunn-Snow, P., & Joy-Smellie, S. (2000). Teaching art therapy techniques: Mask-making, a case in point. *Art Therapy, 17*(2), 125–131. https://doi.org/10.1080/07421656.2000.10129512

Egnell, R., & Alam, M. (Eds.) (2019). *Women and gender perspectives in the military: An International comparison.* Georgetown University Press.

Ferrell, E. L., Russin, S. E., & Grant, J. T. (2021). On being a client with posttraumatic stress disorder: Interactions with treatment providers and institutional barriers. *Journal of Community Psychology, 49*(3), 791–805. https://doi.org/10.1002/jcop.22359

Hourani, L., Williams, J., Bray, R., & Kandel, D. (2014). Gender differences in the expression of PTSD symptoms among active duty military personnel. *Journal of Anxiety Disorders, 29,* 101–108. https://doi.org/10.1016/j.janxdis.2014.11.007

Jones, J. P., Walker, M. S., Drass, J. M., & Kaimal, G. (2018). Art therapy interventions for active duty military service members with post-traumatic stress disorder and traumatic brain injury. *International Journal of Art Therapy, 23*(2), 70–85. https://doi.org/10.1016/j.aip.2019.04.004

Martin, E. G. (2013). Mindfulness practices in art therapy with veterans. *LMU/LLS theses and dissertations, 30.* https://digitalcommons.lmu.edu/etd/30

Oberweis, T., & Bradford, M. (2017). From camouflage to classrooms: An empirical examination of veterans at a regional midwestern university. *The Journal of Continuing Higher Education, 65*(2), 106–114. https://doi.org/10.1080/07377363.2017.1320181

Oppermann, B. (2019). Women and gender in the US military: A slow process of integration. In R. Egnell & M. Alam (Eds.), *Women and gender perspectives in the military: An international comparison* (p. 113). Georgetown University Press.

Smith, A. (2016). A literature review of the therapeutic mechanisms of art therapy for veterans with post-traumatic stress disorder. *International Journal of Art Therapy, 21*(2), 66–74. https://doi.org/10.1080/17454832.2016.1170055

Chapter 17

Healing the Wounds of War

René A. Burgoyne

Basic Training

To establish some background for what soldiers experience, it's necessary to start at the beginning. In this chapter, the term "soldier" is used as a universal term to interchangeably mean Marine, sailor, airman, or Coast Guardsman. Everyone who joins the military has one thing in common: they must swear in by reciting the military oath of enlistment or military oath of office (U.S. Army, 2023). Each soldier swears to defend (not a person) and to accept the orders of the military chain of command. Finally, the soldier vows to face the UCMJ (Uniform Code of Military Justice) should any disputes arise. Once sworn in and entering a specific branch of service, the soldier begins basic training or boot camp. This is where they learn the basics of becoming a soldier. Basic training is designed to be highly intense and challenging. The challenge comes as much from the difficulty of physical training as it does from the psychological adjustment to an unfamiliar way of life. In the end, the soldier learns that there are two basic military functions: waging war and preparing for war. The next step for most is advanced individualized training (AIT). This is a military school where each soldier learns how to do their job while serving. Some schools last for several weeks and others for up to a year. After graduation, they receive orders for their first duty station. In short, some duty stations are deployed to war zones and others are not. Regardless of deployment status, all soldiers are equally trained and ready to go at a moment's notice (U.S. Government Accountability Office Reports, 2009).

Ready for Battle

Battle doesn't begin when a soldier is on the front lines; it starts with preparation and training. Preparation and training include the following: situational awareness, survival training, fitness training, and mindfulness. Simply put, situational awareness is about knowing what is going on in the

DOI: 10.4324/9781003365648-22

environment. Survival training is another step in this process used to teach survival skills or as a form of recreational activity in which individuals are generally challenged to sustain their basic needs, such as food, water, and shelter, in an unpopulated area, with little or only natural resources. Fitness training is exactly what it sounds like, being physically fit. Only the military trains every soldier at a high degree of fitness. As our soldiers get ready to deploy, they must complete a final step which makes deployment quite frightening for most. It's called "Getting your affairs in order." This has become the euphemism of choice for "properly taking care of things before you die." It's where the soldier completes paperwork so if they don't come home alive, the designated loved one will take care of final matters on the soldier's behalf.

Finally, there is the practice of mindfulness. Mindfulness is the basic human ability to be fully present, aware of where we are and what we're doing, and not to be overly reactive or overwhelmed by what's going on around us. For many reasons, the practice of mindfulness can save a life. One of the reasons it can be helpful during deployment is that you're operating on high alert and can become anxious very easily. When you are deployed to an area of the world that you are unfamiliar with, you need to be fully present and aware of where you are and what you are always doing. Otherwise, it could result in a soldier's injury or death.

Wearing a Mask

Soldiers are good at wearing a mask of tenacity and rarely ask for help because they are trained in the same basic manner. They are trained to run toward a firefight, not away. There is no need to ask for help as it is expected that whatever needs to be done will get done. No one ever needs to be told to do something. This was all part of military training and the camaraderie that was established early on during basic training. Despite the myriad of training maneuvers, large-scale exercises, and live-fire exercises... nothing really prepares one for the visceral ugliness of combat. Sometimes this mask of tenacity takes other forms such as addiction, and in others it's in the form of PTSD or both, but either way, the mask serves the veteran to keep them feeling safe. Individuals with PTSD, an anxiety disorder, have typically experienced a traumatic event or exposure to extended periods of stressful or traumatic conditions causing behaviors of hyperarousal, negative mood or cognitive associations, avoidance, and a re-experiencing of the traumatic event (Bahraini et al., 2014). In a phenomenological inquiry of military-related PTSD, Kroch (2009) found several major themes in the experience: trauma remembering; encountering death; hypervigilance in an unsafe world; dualistic psychological ideas (e.g., inner vs. outer worlds, public vs. private life, night vs. day); and feeling alien to oneself and others. I've heard some veterans who are wearing the mask say, "It feels safer that way. Nobody understands what I went through." Difficulty with connection is one of the main difficulties that veterans experience.

According to the *DSM-5* (APA, 2013), post-traumatic stress disorder (PTSD) is included in a new category, trauma- and stressor-related disorders (p. 265). All the conditions included in this classification require exposure to a traumatic or stressful event as a diagnostic criterion. PTSD is the ultimate hidden enemy. It sneaks up on the veteran, never knowing when the ambush will occur. The veteran is on constant alert. The unexpected attacks are brutal, forcing the veteran to relive the unspeakable event(s) again and again. In the book *Tears of a Warrior*, Seahorn and Seahorn (2012) wrote, "If We Send Them, We Must Then Mend Them" (p. 1). They talk about the mass destruction of a battle zone and the effects it has on the body and soul. The first chapter also mentions that the cost of war is rarely talked about. For decades, society failed to encourage people to identify and express emotions. Men and boys were raised not to cry because they'd be "sissies" – "Rub some dirt in it!" or "don't cry over spilled milk." Why is there all this negativity about crying and expressing ourselves? That's what babies do to get their needs met! When did we stop believing that we don't need to get our needs met? It sets one up for confusion and possibly a loss of the sense of self. If we become so disconnected and don't know what we're feeling, how do we know we're alive? Feeling emotions is a basic human condition. It's what separates us from other animals. Society, some families, and the military teach us that emotions are bad. In my opinion, emotions are never good or bad...they just are. Emotions can be helpful, and they can be unhelpful, it just depends on what you do with them. What's most important is having knowledge of what you're feeling, then deciding what to do with that feeling. In the case of being in the throes of battle, emotions can be very unhelpful because they can cause someone to be killed. But in most every other life experience, emotions let us know we're alive. In the book *The Body Keeps the Score*, Vander Kolk (2014) wrote "How do we know we're alive?" (p. 92). He further discusses a study that was done at Harvard Medical School in 1994 that references how the midline structures of the brain don't light up in people who are diagnosed with PTSD as compared to those who aren't. This area of the brain is responsible for emotions and sensations which define terror. Furthermore, with a lack of self-awareness, people with significant PTSD have difficulty recognizing themselves and finding a sense of meaning and purpose in their life. "The structures in charge of self-recognition may be knocked out along with the structures related to self-experience" (Vander Kolk, 2014, p. 94). For those who have experienced trauma, it is often difficult to talk about it in terms of words, since it is imprinted not just as memories but also emotional and physical sensations.

Malchiodi (2020) wrote about the significance of traumatic experiences being encoded within the limbic system and suggested that exteroception (sight, hearing, touch, smell, and taste) and interoception (internal sensations) were foundational to expressive arts and traumatic stress. The expressive arts include interoception in the form of "gut feelings" when referring to the polyvagal system theory (Porges, 2012). Furthermore, expressive arts can help clients to be grounded in the present, stay in the here and now, and take the focus away from past experiences. Healing the wounds of war is not for the faint of heart. It's difficult to hear some of the detailed stories our veterans have experienced. However, it is a privilege to be able to hold space for them to do so. It's easy to ignore the price a warrior pays for our freedom. As an Army veteran serving as a board-certified art therapist at the Veterans Health Administration Mental Health Residential Rehabilitation Treatment Program (MHRRTP), I am honored to share the stories of veterans who continue their battle and find their voice through mask making.

Mask Making

Mask images and therapeutic notes are used to provide a visual and narrative representation of the self as it relates to individual personhood, relationships with others, the community, and society. Imagery themes referenced the injury, relational supports/losses, identity transitions/questions, and conflicted sense of self. As previously mentioned, preparing for war and preparing for battle use the same strategy; therefore my approach with this directive is similar. Situational awareness training is the part of the art therapy session when I orient the veteran to the art studio, the mask making process, and the art materials available. I provide each veteran with a safe space in which they can focus on their inner experience without fear of judgment. The primary goal of the mask making session in the beginning is to provide an opportunity for a veteran to artistically externalize parts of themselves in a safe and non-judgmental environment. Next, I offer them survival training; the survival training is where we work with reinforcing cognitive behavioral therapy (CBT) interventions to give the veteran a sense of agency over any triggers that may surface during the art making process. Fitness training occurs in the art studio as they become acquainted with the art materials, practicing with the materials, mastering the process, and asking for assistance if needed. They are offered a range of art supplies, including paint, collage, and print materials, that enable them to create personal symbols and metaphors within their masks. During this step, asking for assistance with the supplies is the start of learning to interact with and socialize with others and in other areas of their life, which shows tremendous growth. Putting your matters in order is gathering the art media and knowing how to use it and where to obtain what is needed. This is a state of complete independence and total agency over their process. Finally, the act of practicing mindfulness happens throughout the entire process, but especially at the end of the mask making process. When they begin to find their words while looking at their mask, they allow themselves to be vulnerable. Vulnerability takes courage and the veterans have lots of experience being courageous; only now, it extends beyond the uniform. The outside of the mask represents how the world sees them, and the inside of the mask represents how they see themselves. Processing their masks in a group format helps to deepen their understanding of themselves and connect to others. This process helps to regain the camaraderie among each other and the sense of feeling seen and understood.

Psychological Injuries and Challenges

Two main themes presented themselves during the making of the masks: psychological challenges and substance use disorders. Psychological challenges and PTSD symptoms resulting from their military experiences (e.g., an inability to express oneself, addiction, depression, anxiety, and anger) were frequently represented with lips sealed or covered. Substance use disorders often served the service member in dire times, such as during their active-duty service or once discharged, without wanting to admit the need for help.

Case Example: Donny M.

Examples of masks showing psychological injuries and challenges representing: (a) the inability to speak and communicate about traumatic memories exhibited by a false smile or a skeleton hand over the mouth (Figure 17.1a), and (b) the service member's feeling of being "broken," represented through the tears on the inside of the mask along with a significant "loneness" of being empty inside, represented by the white of the inside (Figure 17.1b), as well as the emptiness of the black holes where there once were eyes.

These masks provide examples of psychological injuries represented through color/lack of color, use of line, and facial expressions. The reason for Donny's referral was "to address my PTSD so that I stop drinking… I've been holding it all in, I've got no trust in nobody, and I got no relationships because I start pushing them away or stop communicating with them." Donny stated that he has nightmares related to "a tank firing at us while I was driving in a Jeep. I thought I was dead. After that, I had a hard time throwing a grenade or shooting a rifle. I was in communications in Europe during the Cold War. We were the first ones on the front lines. We were watching the Russians do their military maneuvers." Donny arrived in the art therapy studio each time dressed casually, soft-spoken, and most

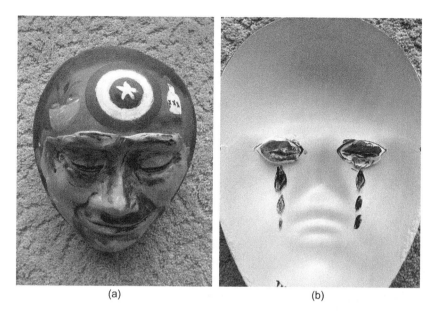

(a)   (b)

Figure 17.1 Donny's masks. Photographed by the author.

Photograph by the author.

often surveyed the area before deciding where to sit. After a few sessions, he determined a spot and claimed it as his own. Donny's mask shows shame on the outside, as represented by the face casting a downward stare. He reports that he's crying because he feels alone in his fear. He said, "Thanks for letting me do this. I'm glad I was able to show you what I've been holding in for so long." The sense of community he felt is seen in the symbolism at the top of the mask. In the center, he puts the symbol for Captain America, which is a superhero. This symbol was flanked by art supplies on the left and alcohol bottles on the right. He said, "I'm an artist and I like to drink." The process of creating the artwork for his mask was soothing and therapeutic for him.

Case Example: Doug H.

In exploring this mask (Figure 17.2), uncertainty regarding current clinical symptoms and future prognosis was evident: (a) the skeleton hand represents questions around his condition and uncertainty about his future, and (b) the third eye represents the service member's feeling that part of him is

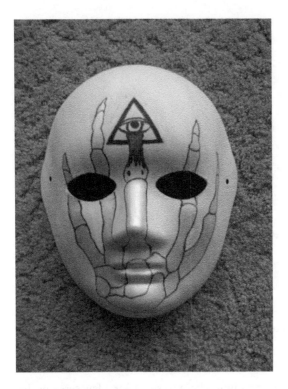

Figure 17.2 Doug's mask.

Photographed by the author.

confused and unsure of his condition while the rest of him is searching for answers.

The reason for Doug's referral was to address his substance use, anxiety disorder, and major depressive disorder. Doug served in the Marine Corps during the Persian Gulf War and when asked about his time in the service he says, "I don't think about the military so much. I don't really know. I hate being told what to do and I hate being on time or early now that I'm done in the military." Statements like these often show how veterans attempt to numb their experiences either through isolation or the use of substances. The transition back to civilian life can be very difficult for some veterans. Doug explained his mask in this way: "The mask I created captures the overwhelming [feeling] of my anxiety. There are times my mind is consumed with death – so much to the point I rush every aspect of my life. I just want to get to the good parts before I go." Doug is struggling with sitting in the uncomfortable messiness of emotions because he will have to feel. Instead of "rushing every aspect of my life," Doug is learning to slow down and be mindful. That is something he has run away from ever since being discharged from the military. Hopefully, one day, Doug will find the courage to face his demons and sit in the uncomfortableness in order to begin to live life on life's terms.

The masks in this chapter refer to emotional struggles around managing overwhelming emotions (e.g., death and sadness represented frequently in shades of "darker" colors and bones of skeletons; explosions referring to anxiety as feeling "consumed"). Symptoms of PTSD (e.g., the inability to articulate what happened) were represented by the mouth being covered or shown with a jester-like grin. Furthermore, engaging in a group art therapy setting provided an opportunity for others suffering with similar feelings the chance to provide positive feedback in a nonjudgmental and safe environment.

Conclusion

Art therapy mask making provides a graphic representation of some of the unseen struggles, challenges, and lived experiences of the service members who have sustained physical and comorbid psychological disorders. This chapter identifies themes in service members' visual representations of the self through masks, including references to psychological injuries, substance use, PTSD, grief, struggles with transitions, and questions about the future. It's important to highlight the lived experience and "unseen" struggles of the service members who have sustained physical and comorbid psychological disorders in this way. This, in turn, offers clinicians at integrative medical care settings an avenue to understand service members' experiences beyond the narrative descriptions alone.

Disclosure Statement

No potential conflict of interest was reported by the author. The views expressed in this chapter are those of the author and do not necessarily reflect the official policy or position of the Department of Veterans Affairs, nor any agency of the US Government. The identification of institutional logos, specific products, does not constitute endorsement or implied endorsement on the part of the author, DoD, Department of Veterans Affairs, or any component agency.

References

American Psychiatric Association (APA). (2013). *Diagnostic and statistical manual of mental disorders*, 5th ed. American Psychiatric Association Publishers.

Bahraini, N. H., Breshears, R. E., Hernández, T. D., Schneider, A. L., Forster, J. E., & Brenner, L. A. (2014). Traumatic brain injury and posttraumatic stress disorder. *Psychiatric Clinics of North America*, *37*(1), 55–75. https://doi.org/10.1016/j.psc.2013.11.00

Kroch, R. (2009). *Living with military-related posttraumatic stress disorder (PTSD): A hermeneutic phenomenological study* [Doctoral thesis]. http://www.collectionscanada.gc.ca/obj/thesescanada/vol2/002/NR54472.PDF

Malchiodi, C. A. (2020). *Trauma and expressive arts therapy: Brain, body, & imagination in the healing process.* Guilford Press.

Porges, S. (2012). *The polyvagal theory.* Norton.

Seahorn, J., & Seahorn, A. (2012). *Tears of a warrior*, 2nd ed. Team Pursuits.

U.S. Army. (2023, March 30). *Oath of enlistment: Oath of office.* https://www.army.mil/values/oath.html

U.S. Government Accountability Office Reports. (2009). *Military personnel: Reserve component servicemembers on average earn more income while activated.* https://www.gao.gov/products/gao-09-688r

Vander Kolk, B. A. (2014). *The body keeps the score.* Penguin.

Chapter 18

Faces Behind the Masks in Times of War

First Aid of the Soul in Ukraine

Nathalie Robelot-Timtchenko

Using the arts allows for a safe container to externalize feelings when life feels uncontainable, especially in times of war. Art making within a group encourages self-expression and employs support through engagement with creativity in a common space (Walker et al., 2017). The emphasis in these groups is on strengths and using themselves and one another as resources. Mask making is a way to understand oneself better, because it offers the opportunity to explore one's identity or hide what may need protection. It is a visual representation of the individual in relation to their community. Engaging in this creative process allows for restored versions of the self to emerge as one copes with and adapts to unimaginable circumstances due to crisis and the brutality of war.

The War Against Ukraine

On February 24, 2022, Russia launched its full-scale invasion against Ukraine, causing an unprecedented act of violence the world has not witnessed since World War II. Tens of thousands of people have been killed, lost their homes, and were forced to flee their country and leave their known lives behind. As of 2023, the estimated number of people requiring humanitarian assistance has reached over 17.6 million, with over six million internally displaced families across the entire country of Ukraine, and over seven million officially registered refugees (Bandura & Reynal, 2023). The ongoing horrors of the war against Ukraine have led to a boundless loss of life, severe injuries, and mass movements of civilians, with over 9,500 killed and more than 16,900 injured (OHCHR, 2023).

Mental Health Challenges in Ukraine

For centuries, Ukraine has had a history of being oppressed, marked by totalitarianism, genocide, mass migrations, and shifting borders. Ukraine's history has a wealth of trauma, collective trauma, and trauma that has

DOI: 10.4324/9781003365648-23

been passed down from generation to generation (Głowacka-Grajper & Wylegała, 2020). Ukraine gained its independence in 1991, yet there is still stigma about seeking mental health support and a lack of funding for services. This is in part due to psychology being used as a weapon throughout the Soviet Union; for example, it was a way to imprison people who had public opinions that differed from the government (Bandura & Reynal, 2023). However, the current First Lady Olena Zelenska has made major strides and efforts addressing the importance of mental health issues, which helped to reduce the stigma that many Ukrainians have had (Presidential Office of Ukraine, 2022).

According to preliminary estimates, more than 15 million Ukrainians have war-related mental health problems and require support for mental exhaustion, bodily injury, and experiences of cruelty (The Ministry of Economy of Ukraine, 2022). In a recent study conducted by the United Nations Development Program (UNDP) in June 2023, they estimated that over 30% of Ukrainians will suffer from more severe health conditions due to post-traumatic experiences of the war, grief and loss, and displacement from their homes (Bandura & Reynal, 2023). The detrimental effects of war trauma for children lead not only to mental health concerns but also may restrict their development physically, cognitively, and relationally. They often develop aggressive or challenging behaviors associated with their trauma which are acted out in their interactions with peers and caregivers (Catani, 2018). Their families continue to live under a prevailing threat of danger daily, in turn preventing them from processing these traumatic events because the events are still ongoing.

The Story of First Aid of the Soul

First Aid of the Soul (FAS) was formed in March 2022 with the mission of providing free and accessible mental health support to Ukrainians affected by the war. A global collective of clinical experts from the expressive arts fields was mobilized to offer trauma-informed mental health and psychosocial support services to Ukrainians through multidimensional and holistic approaches, including providing support groups, supervision, mentorship, training, workshops, and self-help materials. FAS is unique in that the emphasis of support provided is through creative modalities by clinicians in trauma-informed expressive arts. The collective of volunteers integrates art, music, movement, and mindfulness, with the goal of creating a safe space in offering a sense of belonging, connection, empowerment, and ultimately building resilience as well as hope. FAS also prioritizes professional training and support for mental health professionals and frontline workers serving Ukrainians. They experience vicarious trauma, emotional exhaustion, compassion fatigue, burnout, and a lack of support; meanwhile the demand for services far outweighs the available supply of professionals to help those in need (Bandura & Reynal, 2023).

Finding Your Inner Superhero: Workshop 1

In the summer of 2022, Olena Lutsenko, who is my colleague, collaborative partner, and a frequent attendee of many FAS services, along with many psychologists in Kyiv, launched several ongoing arts-based support groups for children and caregivers who have been internally displaced. I was invited to lead a workshop in one of Olena's groups in January 2023. For this particular workshop, I was drawn to the theme of building strength and resilience through mask making. Twelve children from the same class, ages eight and nine, were gathered after school to participate in the workshop. Most of these children were newcomers to the area, having been internally displaced due to the war. Some of the children also came from villages and cities that had been under Russian occupation for several months in the spring of 2022. Many had lost loved ones, their homes, and a sense of normalcy, and others had a parent actively serving in the armed forces.

As the workshop began, the children were welcomed into the space and asked to be seated around the table together (see Figure 18.1). The table was filled with a wide range of art materials: paints, markers, glitter, pastels, scissors, colorful paper, glue, stickers, and more. The children's expressions

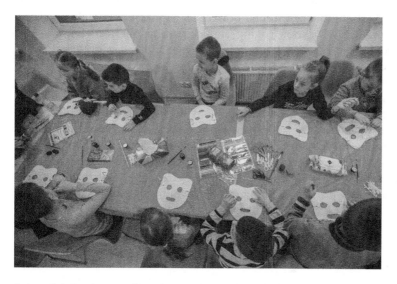

Figure 18.1 The masks and art materials were on the table as we began.
Photograph by New Black Production.

were filled with curiosity and wonder as we got acquainted. Consent was given to film the workshop and take photographs, and the children shared whatever they wanted, depending on their comfort level.

After introductions, the children were invited to share their names and a "super-strength" that they felt represented them. At first, the children were quite shy to engage. I gave a few examples of strengths, a pose, and a sound. Then, one by one, the children began sharing their names and some of their strengths. The schoolteacher and psychologist were extremely helpful in holding a space that was comforting and supportive.

Movement, Rapport, and Safety

Once all the children and adults shared their names and strengths, the children were then invited to play a game in a different area of the room, which required some movement and embodied practices. Starting a therapeutic group with some movement and grounding allows participants to get in touch with their senses and their bodies and to maintain presence within the group. I introduced spectrograms, a psychodrama technique where participants place themselves on a spectrum (range) of where they stand on specific questions. This helps to highlight similarities and differences in comparison with others. This activity created a lot of laughter, bonding, and allowed for the children to be playful with one another and the adults. It was a simple but effective way to build rapport and a sense of safety within the space (Rogers, 1993).

The next grounding directive included some psychoeducation on how to embody strength when feeling powerless. I spoke to the children about the importance of acknowledging and expressing our fears and worries with people who care about us and using one another as resources when those feelings arise (Rogers, 1993). They were then invited to form a circle with or without holding hands. We crouched on the ground, bending our knees, and I asked the children to imagine themselves as a small little plant that is learning how to grow stronger and stronger. This small little plant slowly grows into a large and invincible one because it recognizes its many strengths. As we grew together, moving our bodies from the ground all the way up as high as we could reach and up onto our tiptoes, the infamous champion pose was welcomed into our circle. I shared that the champion pose symbolizes growth and strength and reminded them to try it out on their own when they are sometimes feeling anxious or scared (Staples et al., 2011).

Superhero Mask Making

The group was then guided back to the table. The mask activity was introduced after sharing about my own mask and process. I prompted the children to imagine creating a mask that is filled with their superhero strengths, which could include things they enjoy doing, something they are passionate about, personality traits, their favorite colors, shapes, animals, food, and more. The children were encouraged to enjoy the process of creating and simply playing with the materials and seeing what emerges (Rogers, 1993). Ukrainian music was also played during the workshop. I offered help to the children if they needed it, and one child (who I will call Danya) asked if I could help him draw Spiderman on his mask. The children shared the materials and were patient, calm, friendly, and playful with one another. Another child (who I will call Dima) also asked about drawing Spiderman on his mask. Danya (see Figure 18.2) and Dima chose to use only markers, even when the ink was running low, and persisted in trying to fill their masks with red, using aggressive strokes, rather than using something fluid like paint.

On the other hand, several children using the paint were very gentle with the brushes and moved with precision. Mask themes included animals (e.g., a tiger, colorful cats, a dragon, etc.), superheroes (e.g., Spiderman, Flash, and Sonic), patriotic symbols, and Ukrainian colors. About halfway into the creation process, the electricity shut off, a common occurrence that had been happening around the country to preserve energy during the colder months. However, to my surprise, the children did not react much at all and remained calm. I encouraged them to use the masks as a reminder of their

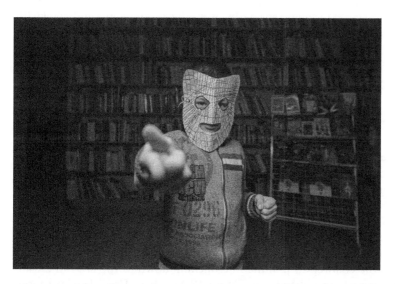

Figure 18.2 This is Danya doing a Spiderman pose with his new mask; notice the markings.

Photograph by New Black Production.

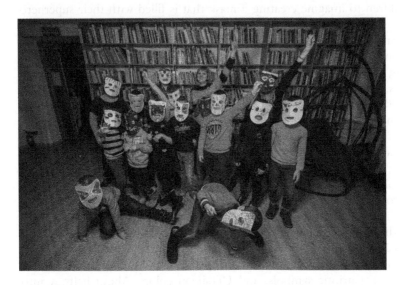

Figure 18.3 The group exploring our superhero power poses.

Photograph by New Black Production.

strength even when things can feel dark. As the children finished working on their masks, they were invited to wear these masks for some group photos and a final directive. The group explored a variety of poses representing different power stances and strengths. It was lively, energetic, and filled with power (see Figure 18.3).

Saying Goodbye

The last part of our time together was, again, with movement, and involved getting back in touch with our bodies (Staples et al., 2011). I brought out a colorful parachute with handles for everyone to grab a hold of. I expressed my sincere gratitude to each of the children and the support staff for allowing me to be with them in the space (see Figure 18.4). As the group gathered around the parachute in a circle, I shared how important it is to have a visual reminder such as a mask to feel a sense of empowerment in times of weakness and that each of them is a superhero and that they all have incredible strength. I reminded them that "It is essential to remember that you are never alone even if sometimes it can feel like it." For our closing ritual, I invited the children to join me in crouching down to the floor in unison with the parachute in hand (see Figure 18.4). Then, I asked them to join me on the count of three, rising up together into our champion poses and releasing the parachute as we rose to the top.

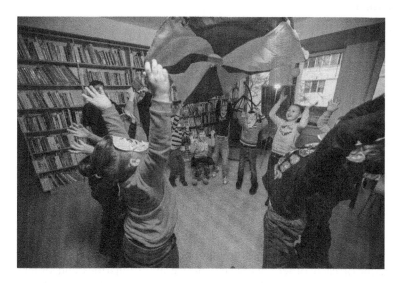

Figure 18.4 The group of children in our final champion pose after releasing the parachute.

Photograph by New Black Production.

As the children left the space, I gave each of them a colorful notebook so they could start creating their individual self-superhero comic books through writing and drawing. I encouraged them to keep sharing their story and to hold onto their strengths. Every child left with their mask on their face and chatting enthusiastically with caregivers about their experience.

Building Resilience: Workshop 2

In the Summer of 2023, there was a series of six two-week residential respite camps being held in a village outside of Kyiv for families coming from a heavily war-affected area in northern Ukraine. FAS was invited to offer several onboarding training courses on various treatment strategies and screening tools for the psychological team that would be facilitating these camps. The training included an overview of psychological first aid, trauma-informed approaches in group work, and expressive arts techniques that support children and teens who are facing severe grief and trauma. In August 2023, I was able to visit these respite camps and also support the team in their work on the ground.

Self-Portraits

After several days of building rapport with the families, I led a workshop on building resilience. As the group began, I introduced myself and spoke about FAS and some of the free-accessible resources and services that are available to them. Lastly, I gave them an overview of the plan for the two-hour workshop and invited them to engage and share their comfort levels. As we started, I asked the group to create a self-portrait using their non-dominant hand and then write down three strengths about themselves. I offered some examples but also invited them to express their portrait in a way that reveals things they like or feel represent them in some way (e.g., nature, music, food, animals, places, style, etc.). Working with the non-dominant hand first helped to relieve potential stress around art making, encourage play, and help the participants feel less judgmental about themselves and their peers (Rogers, 1993). I then led them in some sharing and reflection and asked participants if they felt comfortable raising their images so that everyone could see one another's portraits. I asked them to please be respectful of each other's work and notice any similarities and differences. There were some playful stick figures, lots of nature themes, fashion, favorite animals, foods, and comforting places within the images.

Sharing Strengths

After sharing, I asked the group to please stand and join me in forming a large circle in the center of the room. I brought a ball of yarn and held one piece of it. I invited each participant, parent and child, into our circle to share one strength that they feel is a super-strength of theirs then toss the yarn ball to another while holding their piece of yarn tightly. This directive received many laughs but also engagement from everyone; there was one child who felt too shy to share aloud but still grabbed hold of the yarn alongside her mother. Some of the strengths expressed verbally were family, adaptability, cooking, love, empathy, sports, humor, fashion, animals, and more. I explained the purpose and symbolism behind using the yarn and informed participants that this represents being connected no matter how different we may be. Each of us has our strengths, seen and unseen, and in times of many challenges we need to rely on one another as resources.

Before heading back to the tables, I offered the group the spectrograms game and encouraged them to also ask questions to the group; both the parents and several children took the initiative and participated in leading the game. This brings them back into their bodies and offers a sense of agency within decision-making (Staples et al., 2011). The group was then directed back to the tables for another art directive.

Support and Resources

After a small break, I asked the participants to create another visual of a symbol or sign that represents a support or resource they have drawn upon and will continue to draw upon when facing these ongoing struggles. I also asked them to write down a motto or slogan that would serve as a reminder of that symbol. For this process, I gave the group around fifteen minutes, then opened it up for sharing. One participant (who I will call Karina) was initially reluctant to share but then went first. Karina shared her image of a heart symbol with a Ukrainian flag in the middle. Her slogan said, "Come back alive." She explained that this served as hope that her son and husband would return safely home one day; they are active servicemen. Karina began to cry while sharing, and I asked if the group could offer her and her family a gesture of compassion, using their body. I thanked her for sharing and for her vulnerability, and then we all presented our gestures of support (e.g., heart hands, hands to heart, hugs, victory poses, and strong arms), and she thanked us. A few more participants shared after Karina as well. Some of their resources were family, God, values, nature, music, pets, art, and more. The group was feeling heavy after the sharing, so I offered several breathing and grounding exercises to bring us back into the present and our bodies (Staples et al., 2011).

Strength Mask Making

Then the final directive was introduced: the masks. I emphasized the importance of the mask and that it would serve as a visual reminder of our strengths moving forward. The prompt for the mask making was to create visual symbols or to write their inner strengths down, as well as the strengths and resources they feel they need to rely on more. Finally, I asked them, "What do you need to take with you as a reminder of your strength?" I suggested that they use their previous images and work as inspiration for what to put on their masks. I noticed that most of the words written on the masks were the names of loved ones and values they hold dear. The mask I created (see Figure 18.5) is an example of portraying strength in writing.

As our opening and closing ritual, we gathered once again, standing in a large circle. I placed the yarn back in the center as a reminder of the group connection. As we closed, I asked that each of us share, in order this time, what we are taking with us as a strength from today and a movement that goes along with our mask. As we closed, we counted to three and voiced aloud our strengths in unison.

In Workshop 1, all the children left the room quickly in order to share their experience with their caregivers, but no one stayed to help clean up, given they were not asked to. Meanwhile, in Workshop 2, after every group, not just mine, it was typical for the children and caregivers to clean up

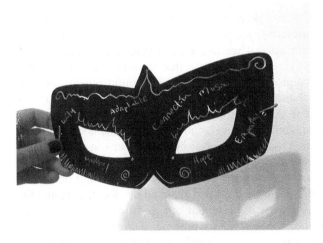

Figure 18.5 The mask I created is an example of portraying strengths in writing.
Photograph by New Black Production.

before leaving. Perhaps, for the participants of Workshop 2, their lives are so chaotic and unknown on a day-to-day basis that keeping order and control wherever and whenever possible is vital.

Conclusion

The people of Ukraine are some of the most resilient individuals I personally and professionally have ever come to know. There is no doubt about their strength, their patriotism, and their willingness to fight for their freedom as a people and as a nation. In times of war, one's sense of meaning, belonging, purpose, and vision for life is shifted to one of survival (Catani, 2018). Expressive arts offer a sense of dignity, respect, and control back to the individual, providing a safe container to explore the meaning and purpose of their life (Rogers, 1993). Restoring an individual's sense of belonging and connection is precisely the mission of First Aid of the Soul. We believe in the power of the healing arts and do our best to execute our work in the most caring and compassionate way. Our ultimate goal is to provide a glimpse of hope and strength to each individual and community we serve.

Acknowledgment

The author would like to thank Olena Lutsenko, who is part of the All-Ukrainian Art Therapy Association in Kyiv, Ukraine, for the continued work she is doing in support of these children and many others.

References

Bandura, R., & Reynal, P. (2023). Investing in mental health will be critical for Ukraine's economic future. Centre for Strategic and International Studies (CSIS), 1–9. https://www.csis.org/analysis/investing-mental-health-will-be-critical-ukraines-economic-future

Catani, C. (2018). Mental health of children living in war zones: A risk and protection perspective. *World Psychiatry, 17*(1), 104–105. https://onlinelibrary.wiley.com/doi/10.1002/wps.20496

Głowacka-Grajper, M., & Wylegała, A. (2020). *The burden of the past: History, memory, and identity in contemporary Ukraine.* Indiana University Press.

Ministry of Economy of Ukraine. (2022, December 9). *Ukraine will build an effective system of providing psychological assistance to preserve the mental health of the nation.* https://www.kmu.gov.ua/news/v-ukraini-pobuduiut-efektyvnu-systemu-nadannia-psykholohichnoi-dopomohy-zarady-zberezhennia-mentalnoho-zdorovia-natsii

OHCHR. (2023, August 14). *Ukraine civilian casualty update.* Office of the UN High Commissioner for Human Rights (OHCHR). https://www.ohchr.org/en/news/2023/08/ukraine-civilian-casualty-update-14-august-2023

Presidential Office of Ukraine. (2022, December 28). *Olena Zelenska told how the initiative to create the national program of mental health and psychosocial support is being implemented.* https://www.president.gov.ua/en/news/olena-zelenska-rozpovila-yak-vtilyuyetsya-iniciativa-zi-stvo-80109

Rogers, N. (1993). *The creative connection: Expressive arts as healing.* Science and Behavior Books.

Staples, J. K., Abdel Atti, J. A., & Gordon, J. S. (2011). Mind-body skills groups for posttraumatic stress disorder and depression symptoms in Palestinian children and adolescents in Gaza. *International Journal of Stress Management, 18*(3), 246–262. https://doi.org/10.1037/a0024015

Walker, M., Kaimal, G., Gonzaga, A., Myers-Coffman, K., & DeGraba, T. (2017). Active-duty military service members' visual representations of PTSD and TBI in masks. *International Journal of Qualitative Studies on Health and Well-Being, 12*(1), 1. https://doi.org/10.1080/17482631.2016.1267317

Chapter 19

Working with Masks in Moscow

A Trauma-Informed Group Narradrama Practice

Ksenia Ilinskaya, Kamran Afary, and Pam Dunne

This chapter presents a case study focused on the narradrama method, examining its application to individuals affected by the collective trauma resulting from the Russian-Ukrainian war. These two nations share a deep cultural bond and an intertwined history. Many families have members who identify as both Ukrainian and Russian, and their relatives and friends have historically maintained mutual relationships. The onset of the war proved to be a profound catastrophe for millions of families in both nations, resulting in a widespread experience of social collective trauma. Among the population of Russia, diverse attitudes towards the war exist, although they are not outwardly expressed through social unrest. The absence of such unrest should not be mistaken as a collective endorsement of the war on Ukraine by the Russian people. Rather, it reveals a deeply ingrained pattern of social silence that has permeated a society shaped by the political dynamics of Russian governments throughout the 20th and 21st centuries. The politics of repression and fear have given rise to an environment where opposition activists are selectively persecuted and openly harassed by supporters of the regime (Gel'man, 2015). This repression has affected individuals from various professions, social statuses, degrees of proximity to the government, and differing opinions, leaving them uncertain about how to avoid persecution.

Repression persisted from the Russian Revolution to the end of the Soviet Union, leading to trans-generational trauma. One generation passed on the experience of inexplicable fear, as countless individuals suffered persecution, instilling fear and anxiety. Almost every family had connections to victims of state persecution. This collective trauma was silently passed down, teaching that remaining invisible is the most effective survival strategy.

As a result, Russians face a current predicament of social trauma, where expressing opinions is challenging, and hope for having a voice is diminished. The oppressive nature of the situation fosters fear, hopelessness, and a sense of powerlessness in effecting meaningful change. Varga and Budinaite (2010) and Varga et al. (2017) assert that Russian society can be characterized as trauma-centric, where each generation remains fixated on the

DOI: 10.4324/9781003365648-24

traumatic experiences endured by previous generations. The primary concern of each generation is to safeguard their children, ensuring their survival and the preservation of the wisdom acquired by those who survived. This wisdom emphasizes isolationist behaviors rooted in fear, such as refraining from collaboration, mistrusting others, and maintaining silence.

Herman (1992, 2023) argues that experiences of abuse disrupt a person's life story, causing it to become chaotic and devoid of meaning. Therefore, the recovery process involves reconnecting the fragmented parts of the story and reconstructing one's self-identity to restore meaning. According to Herman (2023), the process of recovery from trauma comprises three stages:

1. Establishing safety in the present to regain a sense of agency;
2. Revisiting the past, grieving, and making sense of the trauma; and
3. Turning towards the future and forming new relationships with others.

However, Herman emphasizes that therapy alone cannot facilitate the recovery process; it must be intertwined with social processes that contribute to the construction of a social truth (Herman, 2023). According to Hübl (2020), collective trauma entails the suffering experienced by a large number of individuals. Hübl explains that intergenerational trauma, also known as transgenerational, multigenerational, or cross-generational trauma, refers to the consequences of untreated severe trauma passed down from one generation to the next through epigenetic factors. He found that dysfunctional or abusive dynamics within families can persist unaddressed, imprinting implicit messages into the fabric of their identity, thereby posing challenges to the process of creating meaning and purpose in life.

In this chapter, we explore the traumatic experiences of Russians within the context of historical trauma, defined as "cumulative emotional and psychological wounding across generations from massive group trauma experiences" (Maria Yellow Horse Brave Heart, 2003, p. 7). Trauma disrupts connections, leaving individuals isolated and disconnected from their identity, trapped in a narrative of victimhood. Narrative practices shift the focus to seeing the person as a story and trauma as a narrative that perpetuates isolation and shame.

Trauma fractures an individual's life story, dividing their identity before and after the traumatic experience, making them feel disconnected from their skills, resources, and essential aspects of life. To express their experiences and rebuild relationships, individuals must reconnect with their true selves and previous values. Narrative practices encourage exploring the marginalized storyline in responses to trauma, restoring personal agency. Agency involves the belief in influencing their life's trajectory, aligning with their values, and experiencing a responsive world (White, 2016).

By emphasizing the marginalized storyline and renewed agency, individuals can rewrite their identity and redefine their relationship with trauma. An essential part of this process is rediscovering values and deep senses that resonate with their being. White (2000) introduced the term "absent but implicit" to acknowledge that beneath the pain lie essential values distanced from the individual. "Absent but implicit" empowers individuals to transition from anguish to reconnecting with values defining their life's purpose, guiding them towards a preferred identity embodying these cherished values.

The narradrama approach (Dunne et al., 2020) encourages individuals to rewrite life stories into preferred narratives, fostering emotional expression and artistic embodiment. Masks, external representations of preferred identities, facilitate exploration through role-playing, allowing the expression of feelings, attitudes, and physicality. This process empowers individuals to develop new coping strategies based on their preferred values, beliefs, and intentions, shifting their relationship with trauma.

Narradrama offers embodied modalities for expressing trauma's impact when words fall short. It allows expression even when verbal communication is inaccessible or when there is a disconnection with the body due to repression. By incorporating masks and other artistic forms, narradrama engages with the body and offers alternative modes of communication, creating a unique language beyond verbal discourse. Drawings, masks, and sculptures enable diverse individualized expressions, particularly for those suppressed by societal norms and linguistic limitations.

Narradrama Group

A narradrama group was formed in December 2022, a few months after a mobilization that profoundly shocked every family in Russia. Following a period of shock and crucial decision-making (regarding leaving the country, remaining in the country, or finding a safe place to reside), the opportunity for psychotherapeutic work emerged to address social trauma among Russian participants. The group consisted of 11 participants, including one man and ten women, ranging in age from 19 to 55 years old. The group held four meetings, with two sessions per week conducted via Zoom in the evening. Participation in the group was free of charge. Prior to the sessions, participants were informed that the group's description would be included in this chapter, and they provided written consent for their information to be used publicly. Some participants had relocated to other countries, while others remained in Russia for various reasons. Each participant had independently decided to seek assistance in coping with their current situation.

Before describing our meetings, it's crucial to highlight key factors that significantly impacted our group.

- Safety: While addressing trauma typically emphasizes creating a safe environment, our situation lacked this luxury. Families involved in the conflict and restrictions like avoiding the term "war" complicated matters.
- Facilitator's shared trauma: Unlike traditional trauma facilitators, our facilitator shared the same traumatic experiences and shock as participants, affecting the group dynamics.

The group's creation was inspired by narrative practice, emphasizing that everyone can be the author of their own life regardless of circumstances. It underscores recognizing and staying connected with values, the power of identity construction, and rewriting one's life story.

Meeting 1

The first meeting focused on creating an atmosphere of support and safety for participants to express themselves, share their stories, become acquainted with the experiences of others, and make their current situations visible. It was the longest meeting, and it was decided, in consultation with the participants, to extend its duration to three hours in order to ensure that everyone had an opportunity to be heard. The meeting began with a warm-up activity called "What I like to do is... When I'm doing that, I'm like this," where participants expressed themselves through poses, connecting with their interests and preferred selves in a nonverbal manner. The second warm-up activity involved participants choosing an internet picture that resonated with their inner vision of the world before the current events. They were then asked to pose themselves in that imagined situation. The central activity of the meeting involved participants drawing a picture representing their current life situation as they felt it.

After completing their drawings, participants received further instructions:

- They were asked to make their values visible in the picture – those aspects they had managed to hold onto, something they had cherished before and still highly valued, despite the challenges.
- They were instructed to replace something from their previous picture with an element representing their life before the events – selecting parts or shapes that still encompassed their pre-existing identity.
- Participants were encouraged to carefully examine their pictures and identify something hiding behind that was of great importance to them, applying the concept of the "absent but implicit" in a narradrama art therapeutic approach.

Upon finishing their drawings, participants were invited to pose themselves in a way that expressed the importance of their situation. Each participant had the opportunity to share their drawing, express their thoughts, and receive support from the group.

Many participants expressed feelings of silence, loss of connection, and isolation from something deeply important in their lives. For the closing ritual, participants used gestures to show what they would like to give as a gift to other participants.

Meeting 2

The second meeting aimed to deepen participants' understanding of their values and life aspects. It encouraged them to recognize personal needs, separate from societal influences, and make decisions based on their values. This approach, rooted in narrative practice, utilized masks through the narradrama method to help individuals connect with significant life aspects.

Externalizing these aspects allowed for a stronger connection and emotional resonance. The narradrama approach facilitated not only logical understanding but also emotional alignment with personal values to guide one's life story.

The meeting began with participants sharing their impressions from the previous session and expressing current feelings through gestures and sounds. The central activity involved creating masks to represent internal support and embodying their chosen hero's character, exploring movements and behaviors. After this individual exploration, participants formed small groups of three or four people to discuss the answers to the following questions from the perspective of their heroes:

* Where do I live?
* What do I want?
* What is my history?
* What do I stand for?
* What is important to me?

Following the discussion, participants came together to perform collectively, acting as their heroes. Here are some examples of masks and the stories behind them:

* I am Avatar (see Figure 19.1). I have existed for millions of years. I live in high mountains where nature is vibrant and beautiful. Everyone in my world flies on magnificent dragons, with whom they share a special bond. While the world is glorious, there are also many challenges. I fly and observe from different perspectives, fearlessly defending my dragon and being vocal about what I witness.

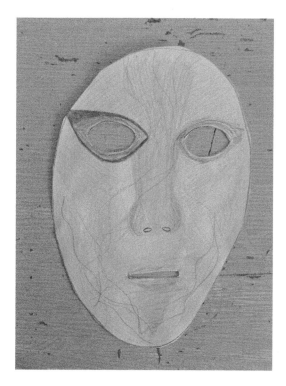

Figure 19.1 Mask of Avatar.

Photograph by Ksenia Ilinskaya.

- I am Togetherness (see Figure 19.2). I have lived alongside humanity since the beginning of time. My purpose is to promote kindness and unity among people. I stand for peace in the world and believe that supporting one another is the only way to survive.

Following discussions, participants delivered captivating performances. One depicted making and enjoying coffee with cardamom and saffron, featuring characters like Seed, Humanity, Togetherness, and Happiness. The second focused on being true to oneself, with characters like Freedom-to-be-Yourself, Equilibrium, and Silence engaging in dialogue. The third showcased a meeting between the Hussar, Avatar, and the Princess of Elves, encountering a dragon and embarking on a journey with elven music, symbolizing aspirations for freedom, connection, and a proactive future.

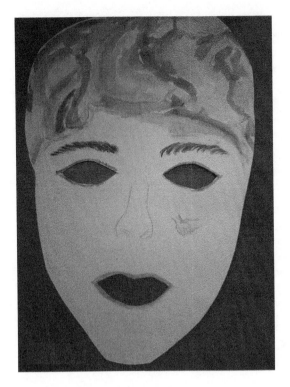

Figure 19.2 Mask of Togetherness.
Photograph by Ksenia Ilinskaya.

To foster group closeness, a brief meeting reflection was followed by a ritual where participants made symbolic gestures to represent the session's impact on each person.

Meeting 3

The third meeting began with a discussion about the previous session and the time that had passed since then. As a warm-up exercise, the narradrama approach incorporated music for externalization. Participants were asked to select music that resonated with their masked character and to move or dance as the character would. The music helped participants connect with their preferred identity, which emerged after wearing the mask, on a bodily level. These movements were intended to help overcome the freezing effect of trauma. Following the dance with the mask, participants sat down and answered the following questions:

- Dear Mask, how long have you been a part of (the author of the mask)'s life?
- How did you become acquainted with (the author of the mask)?
- What do you enable (the author of the mask) to do in life?
- What do you want for them?
- What becomes possible in their life because of your presence?
- What do you think is important to tell them now?

After answering these questions, the participants were asked to prepare a gift for the author of their mask. Subsequently, participants performed monologues as their mask, incorporating their answers to the questions. Following each performance, the other participants engaged in witnessing, selecting the most comfortable mode of expression for them. Three types of witnessing were available:

- Using words: Participants chose three or more words that resonated with what they had seen and heard.
- Using drawing: Participants created an image that connected with what they had witnessed.
- Using gesture: Participants demonstrated a gesture that reflected what they had witnessed.

Regardless of the chosen mode of expression, the focus of witnessing was on the appearance and depth of the preferred story and the reflection of the preferred identity. Examples of monologues:

- Togetherness: I have existed in this world for many years, but I entered (the author of the mask)'s life a few years ago. She experienced the loss of her father and husband, which made her more isolated. With the onset of war, her anxiety increased, and her ability to communicate with others deteriorated. She realized the value of human connections. I entered her life to encourage her to be more open and to communicate more. I offer support and warmth. The words I want to tell her are from a Russian folk saying: Hold onto each other, fear nothing. I want to present her with a scarf, like a life-saving tool from fairy tales. It can provide comfort and warmth, serve as a resting place, shield against the cold, or offer warmth to those close to her. The possibilities are endless!
- Avatar: No one helped us find each other; we did it ourselves. I help her see the beauty in life and be an explorer. I want her to pursue activities that bring her pleasure, and I assist her in doing what she desires more effortlessly. I want to tell her, "Just do what you want to do. Everything is easier than you imagine." I would like to give her a compass.

The meeting concluded with a reflection on the session and a ritual of exchanging gifts among the participants expressed through a virtual gesture.

Meeting 4

The group's warm-up involved a brief discussion and expressing current emotions through gestures. Participants who hadn't presented their previous monologues were invited to do so.

The next step included reflecting on past activities. Participants connected their life situation drawings with their masks, exploring the relationship between the mask and the world. After some action, they spent a minute in introspection, selecting a resonating word or phrase to contribute to a collective poem created by the entire group.

Comfort consists of some distance
You can always find support within yourself
Support
A new dance to new music
When you feel you can lean on something, energy emerges
Do not forget: to let something emerge, you must let go of something else
Go to the forest! You will encounter different things!
Do not forget where you are, where your soul resides.
If you never venture, you will never truly live
Allow me to give you a hug before you go.
Safety and core.

After the sessions were over, participants shared some of their takeaways from this work:

- I feel a great sense of relief. My thoughts were wandering, but now I have a more conscious and precise understanding of my situation, intentions, and aspirations. I feel like I have a plan.
- Thanks to the group, I feel more confident about my position, and it helps me move forward.
- I realized how important balance is for me and how I need more of it right now. I connected with the character, and it was important for me to understand it better.
- For me, this group was a gift that allowed me to focus on myself, which is crucial at the moment. It provided a safe space to express feelings about difficult and painful matters. In the outside world, you have to keep a lot inside due to politics and the suffering of everyone around you. It was wonderful to have a gentle space to touch on all of that, to cry about something, feel joy about something else, let go, and move forward. We

are all journeying through what seems like a dead forest, but we continue together, and nobody is alone.

• Thanks to the Mask, I turned to the spirit and ideas of my character. It enabled me to continue my work here and find answers to my questions about helping others while supporting myself. My picture has transformed slightly. I now see more flowers, and the crack is not as significant as it was before. My character is so beautiful to me that I feel there is much I can learn from them as I move forward.

In conclusion, narradrama provided a gentle way for participants to engage with traumatic experiences, helping them connect with values and abilities to transform their relationship with the inner image of trauma. Lessons from using masks with the narradrama approach in this workshop series include:

• Masks reveal a source of internal support, allowing participants to think, feel, and act from that perspective.
• Through dialogue, reflection, and witnessing, participants can connect with alternative stories and reshape their identities based on their senses.
• Masks offer distance from overwhelming problem stories, helping construct relationships between traumatic situations and alternative narratives.
• Using masks allows exploration of different life areas, shifting from a mono-historical to a poly-historical perspective, empowering participants as authors of their life stories.
• Choosing one's identity in the face of social cataclysm empowers individuals, shifting them from a victim mindset to an active position.
• Utilizing masks can be crucial in resisting trauma's effects and unconscious reactions of fight, flight, or freeze.

References

Dunne, P., Afary, K., & Paulson, P. (2020). Narradrama. In D. R. Johnson & R. Emunah (Eds.), *Current approaches in drama therapy* (pp. 207–304). Charles C Thomas Publishing.

Gel'man, V. (2015). The politics of fear: How the Russian regime confronts its opponents. *Russian Politics and Law, 53*(5–6), 6–26. https://doi.org/10.1080/10611940.2015.1146058

Herman, J. L. (1992). *Trauma and recovery: The aftermath of violence - From domestic abuse to political terror.* Basic Books.

Herman, J. L. (2023). *Truth and repair: How trauma survivors envision justice.* Basic Books.

Hübl, T. (2020). *Healing collective trauma: A process integrating our intergenerational and cultural wounds.* Sounds True Incorporated.

Remarque, E. M. (1929). *All quiet on the western front* (A. W. Wheen, Trans.). Little, Brown and Company.

Varga, A. Y., & Budinaite, G. L. (2010). *The traumas of the past in Russia and the possibilities of applying systemic family psychotherapy.* https://psyjournal.ru /articles/travma-proshlogo-v-rossii-i-vozmozhnosti-primeneniya-sistemnoy -semeynoy-terapii

Varga, A. Ya., Markitanova, O. A., & Cherepanova, E. (2017). *Rules of surviving: The message to children.* https://familypsychology.ru/research/family-survival -rules

White, M. (2000). *Reflections on narrative practice: Interviews & Essays.* Dulwich Centre Publications.

White, M. (2016). *Narrative therapy classics.* Dulwich Center Publications.

Yellow Horse Brave Heart, M. (2003). The historical trauma response among Natives and its relationship with substance abuse: A Lakota illustration. *Journal of Psychoactive Drugs, 35*(1), 7–13. https://doi.org/10.1080/02791072.2003 .10399988

Part V

From Protection to Healing

Chapter 20

Mask Making as a Featured Process in a Hospital-Based Open Studio

Jill McNutt, Erin Hein, and Jane Carriere

Historically, masks have been created with a wide variety of materials, including natural found objects like shells, stones, and feathers, harvested objects like wood, fibers, metals, and clay, animal products like ivory, horns, and leather, and vegetation items like flowers, corn husks, and bark. Ornamentation and finishing have varied from simple feature additions to elaborate additions of jewels and tilework to establish importance (Wingert, 2020). Intentions of masks have included, but are not limited to, memories of persons past, transformations of the spiritual dimension, depiction of stories and characters, and reflecting on the difference between self-perception and self-presentation. The duality of self and other presentation is often accomplished by using two sides of a mask, one side depicting self-perception and the other side depicting presentation to others (Dunn-Snow & Joy-Smellie, 2000). The mask can serve as a form of communication between aspects of the self.

The process of developing masks as artworks has supported the exploration of conscious and/or subconscious personas (Trepal-Wollenzier & Wester, 2002). Mask making facilitates a sense of inner play, promoting self-dialogue and allowing the development of identification, personal protection, and ultimately opportunities for growth (Dunn-Snow & Joy-Smellie, 2000). Mask making often appears as a celebration, masquerade, and is also associated with holidays including but not limited to Día de los Muertos, Halloween, Mardi Gras, and New Year's Eve. Masks have also historically represented supernatural beings, ancestors, or imagined figures (Wingert, 2020).

Open Art Therapy Studio

Open studio as a group format is humanistic in nature (Keleman & Shamri-Zeevi, 2022). The process is meant to flow and adapt to the needs of participants and their interpretation of the art processes used. Purported benefits of open studios facilitated by art therapists include improvement of positive

DOI: 10.4324/9781003365648-26

affect, self-efficacy, and creative energy (Kaimal et al., 2017). Altruism, reparative relationships, and enhancement of neuroplasticity have also been seen as positive results from participation in art therapist-facilitated open studios (Keleman & Shamri-Zeevi, 2022).

The open art therapy studio at Advocate Aurora Health runs four hours twice a month. It has both in-person and virtual components. Participants include patients, former patients, community members, and healthcare workers. Participants can arrive and depart according to their own availability and desires. Some participants stay for the whole time and others come and go throughout the course. Each studio is facilitated by credentialed art therapists who often engage in artmaking alongside studio participants. Teoli (2020) called the act of the client and art therapist creating art simultaneously *companioning artmaking*. Companioning artmaking has been seen to support clients (Hyland-Moon, 2015) and diffuse the power inequality that often exists between clients and mental health professionals (Furneaux-Blick, 2019).

The dynamics of masks in healthcare settings have been accentuated due to the COVID-19 pandemic. At the time when these three studio sessions occurred, it had been less than a year since the COVID-19 restrictions were lifted, and in-person studio attendance resumed. In-person participants are required to wear protective masks during the open studio. Recurring studio participants have reported a variety of healthcare diagnoses including cancer, cardiovascular disease and stroke, cerebral palsy and spina bifida, anxiety and depression resulting from medical conditions, traumatic brain injury, dissociative identity disorder, seizure disorders, and eating disorders.

Featured Process

Each studio session begins with a featured process designed to be specific enough for newcomers to easily engage in the creative process, and open enough for returning participants to expand or embellish the design. Aside from the featured process, the studio is equipped with a wide array of art supplies so that participants may choose any available process. Due to the medical setting, chalk pastels, wet clay, oil-based and aerosol media, and noisy processes that include blenders or other motorized tools have been excluded from the supply carts.

The featured process during the three sessions discussed in this chapter focused specifically on mask making. The three-week process was divided into planning, creating, and interacting with the masks. Each session, instructions were sent to virtual participants ahead of time, and in-person attendees received instructions upon arrival. There were various levels of participation. Some only came to one or two sessions, and some participated in alternate creative processes. The occurrence of the open studios featuring mask making was within six weeks of Halloween.

Mask Makers

Participants who engaged in mask making will be referred to as *mask makers* from this point forward. Over the course of the three open studio sessions, there were 15 mask makers, and three art therapists who served as facilitators in virtual and in-person sessions. The age range of mask makers was ten to 70 years. Participants who did not engage in mask making had ongoing processes to engage in. One participant engaged in an ongoing card-making process, and a second participant worked on an assemblage she had started weeks earlier. Mask makers who attended virtually did so due to lingering ramifications of COVID-19, transportation issues, geographic distance, and personal responsibilities at home. Mask makers came to the open studio as individuals, as families, and as dyads or triads of friends.

At the in-person location, supplies were laid out to support ease of access. Supplies included plaster gauze, model magic, found objects, natural objects, feathers, mask molds, beads, and other embellishments. In-person mask makers collected items from the material display tables, and virtual participants collected materials ahead of time and brought them to open studio sessions. The virtual portion of these open studios was held through a Zoom platform using a laptop computer, and both in-person and virtual sessions ran simultaneously. Art therapists were present in both virtual and in-person formats.

Mask makers engaged with varying levels of imagination and physical and/or developmental ability. Some were more concrete in their expression, while others were more abstract. Some masks were two-dimensional and others were three-dimensional. Masks created during these open studios that featured mask making reflected culture in sports participation and local holiday celebrations, and representations of disguises like witches or fairy-like beings.

Origins of this Report

The information for this report was derived from observations taken during the open studio sessions by each of the three facilitators. As facilitators, we were also companioning the group by creating our own masks alongside the mask makers. After each session, we took notes on the things that we had observed, such as how mask makers interacted with the materials provided, their interactions amongst each other, their interactions with the masks themselves, and our experiences among the mask makers. In addition to these notes, we also drew from mask makers' comments, stories, and the post-group emails that they shared with facilitators. All three art therapists then met to discuss and compare notes. The information from the notes was collected and reviewed to establish the presented themes.

When comparing our observations, we met virtually while working together in a shared document. All observational notes and stories were brought together into this shared document, where we read through the notes and highlighted certain sections that seemed to be related to each other. From these relations, we were able to identify the themes and commonalities. Throughout the meetings, insightful reflection led to an expansion of our understanding of mask making as a featured process in the open studio. From this process, we identified the following themes: materials used, process of engagement, investment in the process, metaphors and archetypes, and the therapeutic value of mask making.

Materials Used

The featured process directive was open-ended in material usage. It included recommendations for collage use and sketching to determine starting points. Many mask makers did engage in brainstorming and sketching processes at the start. Scribbling and digital art media were also primarily used by virtual participants. These preliminary processes were sufficient for some mask makers whose final products remained two-dimensional. The creation of the foundation for masks also took many forms. Papier-mâché, soft clay, plaster gauze, tree bark, aluminum foil, recycled containers, and varieties of tape were sometimes used sometimes around a mold. Some foundations were planned and followed specific designs, while others built upon themselves, and the final shape evolved over time.

Embellishments and finishing layers of the masks used varying levels of intentionality and experimentation. Paint was a common first layer of designs. Feathers, paper flowers, silk flowers, leaves, and stems, fabric, glitter/glitter glue, crystals, beads, sequins, wood, and buttons were among the materials. Trial and error were common and at times left the sentiment of, "next time I would do x, y, and z differently" (see Figure 20.1).

The creator of this mask shared:

I had tried to show closed eyes with the paint line, but it doesn't really read like that. I wish I had done something more three dimensional for the eyes. It's hard to see that it is actually a face shape since I chose to leave off the bottom portion of the mask. Next time, I might exaggerate the facial features more to help them show up.

Process of Engagement

Drawing and two-dimensional art processes were a component of the mask-making sessions. Several people sketched their masks initially as instructed

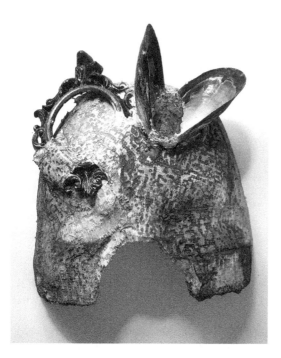

Figure 20.1 Inner thoughts mask.

Photographed by the creator.

in the first dedicated mask session. One participant enjoyed this process so much that he sketched a variety of masks each session. Limitations directed a two-dimensional mask making process for at least two participants. One in-person participant was limited by an unspecified disability, and one virtual participant was limited by materials available at home. The two-dimensional masks were cut from paper and used string to tie behind the head. Two-dimensional mask drawings included scribbles, designed sports logos, and visual storytelling.

Three-dimensional mask making processes included gathering supplies, experimentation with materials, adaptations, and some mask makers used preformed plastic molds. Some supplies were gathered from within the material collection of the studio itself, others were collected from outdoors and mask maker's homes. Mask makers experimented with foundational materials in creating the basic forms of the mask while adapting processes dependent on aesthetic choice. Variations in form included real and imaginary features. One mask maker created masks out of aluminum foil, painted

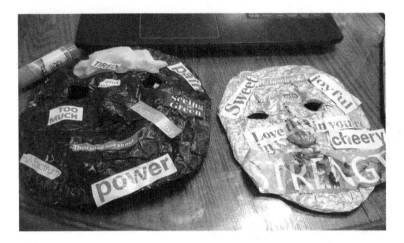

Figure 20.2 Disability mask.

Photograph by the creator.

them and embellished using words cut from magazines (see Figure 20.2). These masks "show how I feel about my disability from the inside and what I show to others."

Mask design and decoration were sometimes done in a trial-and-error method, and were often completed with focused intention. Embellishments were added through the use of hot glue and other adhesives to help accomplish the mask maker's goal. Mask maker goals included cultural aspects, realistic and exaggerated facial expressions, and representations of personality and persona.

Investment in Process

Mask makers came at various times throughout the sessions. Each took some time to get into a creative headspace, then seemed to become more invested in the process. Some mask makers were more serious, some more playful. Mask makers were interested, invested time with the use of collage and sketching, and engaged while working on their mask projects. For some, there were moments that became cumbersome and required some problem solving. These times created quiet and deliberate engagement. Those who found challenging moments engaged deeply. One virtual mask maker identified closed eyes and a closed mouth in her mask depiction. This mask maker shared, "I cannot see, and how can I advocate for myself if I cannot speak?"

The further mask makers got into their process, playfulness and experimentation became more prevalent. No matter how much time a mask maker had to invest, all were able to engage fluently while working. One young mask maker was so engaged that he remarked, "I didn't know I could have this much fun without a Nintendo Switch." Sometimes the experimentation led to discoveries like surprise and excitement over sequins melting in hot glue, "it's melting – my pretty," or the ability of Model Magic to create facial features, "it's magic! It's sticking!"

Families who came together both engaged individually and provided support as a family unit. Mothers checked in frequently with children (both adult children and youth), sometimes aiding in the process, and other times offering encouragement. One facilitator worked individually with an adult male with a cognitive disability who required constant support and a working third hand to create his masks. The "third hand" is a concept in art therapy that refers to the connection between the art therapist, client, and the art materials used (Moon, 1990). The art therapist became an extension of this mask maker. The mother and sister repeatedly looked up to check in on the adult male.

Several participants conceptualized the idea of masks before the groups started. Following planning, participants took it upon themselves to collect materials outside of sessions. Some even started building their masks before returning to the second or third session. A couple of participants completed their masks at home and brought them in to share with the group (see Figure 20.3). Overall, there was satisfaction with the masks created during these three sessions.

The creator of this mask shared:

"These photos represent the evolution of a single sketch that I did then and the photographically embellished morphs that followed. The premise was a depiction of myself as an owl showing the healing process."

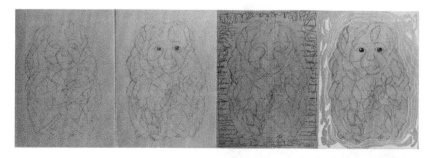

Figure 20.3 Scribble mask progression.
Photograph by the creator.

Metaphors and Archetypes

Elements of the masks and expressions regarding the masks echoed real-life experience. Portions of masks were referred to as commentary on life events. The mannerisms of mask sharers portrayed significant aspects of personality, trauma, and symptoms of conditions or states of mind. Some masks highlighted the physical realities of the mask makers. Elements of pain, choking away voice and/or breath, tension in the neck and other muscular areas were present. Some masks that were created with a sense of play felt more relaxed. One mask included a limited version of facial covering, perhaps indicative of a distaste for facial coverings conflicting with wearing glasses (see Figure 20.4).

The creator of this mask shared:

> Currently, it is more of a tiara than a mask. It turned out almost exactly like I had drawn it. It feels very ethereal. I feel like leaving the face section more open, partially due to my glasses, but also as a way to say that I'm allowing my actual self to show through the strongest, my inner goddess is being shown and encouraged.

Some mask makers intentionally used colors to represent factors of their own life experiences. These colors were said to represent trauma, personas of varying demographics, cultural celebrations, and personal expression preferences. Rainbow colors were used to represent respect and inclusion of LGBTQIA+. Symbolism was prevalent in the work of mask makers in

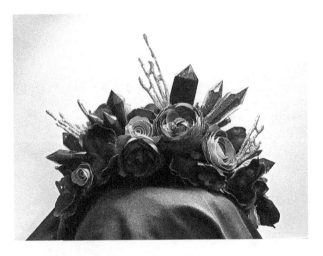

Figure 20.4 Goddess mask.

Photograph by the creator.

both conscious and subconscious expression. One mask maker identified with an image of an owl and created the mask in the form of that image. A peacock was used to express spreading wings and appreciating accomplishment. Another mask maker intentionally used hearts on the cheek of the mask as a symbol of love, compassion, and joy. Personas present in the masks included fortune tellers/clairvoyants, demons or witches, royalty, and inner goddesses. Elements were described as ethereal, mystic, and natural.

Therapeutic Value of Mask Making

The therapeutic value of mask making was apparent in self-expression, stress relief, emotional expression including both celebratory and traumatic catharsis, and processing mental capacity. Participants played with how to wear their individual masks, how much of their face to leave exposed, and how much to keep hidden. Contemplations included cultural elements including holidays, sports enthusiasm, and personal affirmations of strength and accomplishments. One mask maker discussed no longer resonating with an artificial smile and recognized several symbols of personal growth. Another mask maker accidentally broke the clay mask and had thoughts on a changing life due to illness, a cathartic break, or a "difficult stress fracture" (Figure 20.5).

Participants actively engaged in processing both emotions and mental capacity. This was done while brainstorming, using collage, engaging symbolically with found objects, dialogue, and witnessing. Outside stressors seemed to recede while participants engaged in collecting materials, building masks, and engaging with facilitators. The body language of some participants visibly relaxed over the duration of the studio time, and verbally discussing mask components allowed the cathartic release of stress and tension. The atmosphere within the studio space was frequently filled with laughter and playful chatter. The masks created a sense of playfulness and belonging for each of the mask makers.

Looking Back

Mask makers engaged as deeply as they wished without needing to be encouraged to do so. A natural process of engagement typically occurs within open studios in this setting. The extended focus on masks helped mask makers to carry on between sessions; this highlighted the engagement and reduced the need for a warm-up process for those who came already engaged.

The flexibility of timing, wide variety of materials, and openness to the project facilitated mask makers' ability to ground the experience in current states of mind. This flexibility also led to realistic expectations and honored

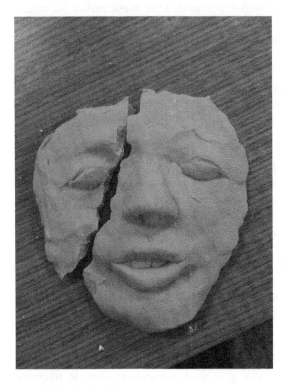

Figure 20.5 Broken Mask.
Photograph by the creator.

diversity as the masks were completed. The studio allowed enough freedom for people to express themselves as necessary.

When planning this sequence of studios in the future, plans might include the addition of sharing elements where each mask maker would have the opportunity to share the process, image, and potential meaning of the masks with the entire group. Other options would include having sessions weekly instead of biweekly and bringing materials as part of the instruction for in-person attendees to encourage continuous participation. Mask makers who attended online reported feeling left out of smaller group communications during the art making process. Separating the virtual sessions from the in-person sessions may provide a more consistent platform and eliminate awkward collaboration between virtual and in-person mask makers. Overall, the three-mask making open studio sessions were a success.

References

Dunn-Snow, P., & Joy-Smellie, S. (2000). Teaching art therapy techniques: Mask-making, a case in point. *Art Therapy, 17*(2), 123–131. https://doi.org/10.1080/07421656.2000.10129512

Furneaux-Blick, S. (2019). Painting together: How joint activity reinforces the therapeutic relationship with a young person with learning disabilities. *International Journal of Art Therapy, 24*(4), 169–180. https://doi.org/10.1080/17454832.2019.1677732

Hyland-Moon, C. (2015). Open studio approach to art therapy. In D. E. Gussak & M. L. Rosal (Eds.), *The Wiley handbook of art therapy* (pp. 112–121). Wiley Blackwell. https://doi.org/10.1002/9781118306543

Kaimal, G., Mensinger, J. L., Drass, J. M., & Dieterich-Hartwell, R. M. (2017). Art therapist-facilitated open studio versus coloring: Differences in outcomes of affect, stress, creative agency, and self-efficacy (Studio ouvert animé par un art-thérapeute versus coloriage : Différences de résultats sur l'affect, le stress, l'agentivité créatrice et l'efficacité personnelle). *Canadian Art Therapy Association Journal, 30*(2), 56–68. http://doi.org/10.1080/08322473.2017.1375827

Keleman, L. J., & Shamri-Zeevi, L. (2022). Art therapy open studio and teen identity development: Helping adolescents recover from mental health conditions. *Children, 9*(7), 1029. https://doi.org/10.3390/children9071029

Moon, B. L. (1990). Third hand: Collaboration in art therapy. *The Arts in Psychotherapy, 17*(4), 309–316.

Teoli, L. (2020). Art therapists' perceptions of what happens when they create art alongside their clients in the practice of group therapy. *The Arts in Psychotherapy, 68*, 1–24. https://doi.org/10.1016/j.aip.2020.101645

Trepal-Wollenzier, H. C., & Wester, K. L. (2002). The use of masks in counseling: Creating reflective space. *Journal of Clinical Activities, Assignments and Handouts in Psychotherapy Practice, 2*(2), 123–130. https://doi.org/10.1300/J182v02n02_13

Wingert, P. S. (2020). *Encyclopedia Britannica*. https://www.britannica.com/art/mask-face-covering

Chapter 21

The Transformation of a Radiation Mask

Susan Ridley and Terri Giller-Etheridge

Both Susan Ridley and Terri Giller-Etheridge have taught the undergraduate introduction to creative arts therapy course to students at West Liberty University in West Virginia, USA. The course provides an opportunity for them to explore the variety of ways that the arts are used in therapy. Students learn about the history of art therapy and the early pioneers of the profession, the influence of Indigenous healing practices, and psychological theory. Additionally, this class explores various populations and settings in which art therapy currently provides benefits and discusses the future of the field. An important aspect of this course, however, is the experiential opportunities for students to engage in art making and reflection on the creative process, which helps to promote personal insight as an artist.

Archetype Masks

At the beginning of the 16-week course, students learn about Jung's theory of archetypes and are given the assignment to create an archetype mask. Carl Jung used the term "archetypes" when describing the fundamental, universal symbols and themes that make up the instinctual energy in the human psyche (Jung, 1969). According to Jung, archetypes are recurring patterns of behavior that exist across cultures and time periods, originating from the collective unconscious (Swan-Foster, 2018). To put it simply, these archetypes are the building blocks that shape how individuals interact with and perceive the world. Early on, Jung identified four major archetypes – the "persona," "anima/animus," "shadow," and "self." Jung went on to write that there are no limits to the number of archetypal motifs that can be seen in myths, stories, religious texts, and art from various cultures and time periods. These include "the creator," "the explorer," "the lover," "the hero," etc.

When choosing an archetype to explore, students consider their own personal identity, journey, and/or aspirations. Students are asked to identify one or more archetypes that best represent how they view themselves.

DOI: 10.4324/9781003365648-27

During their research on their chosen archetype(s), students identify examples throughout history and in the arts/culture for the written paper component of the assignment. Students are offered a choice of using a mask form, creating their own, or creating a plaster cast of their face using plaster rolls. Materials range from papier-mâché, plaster, cardboard, to found objects. Students may choose a form and then paint the mask, collage paper, or fabric, or add embellishments such as natural items, glitter, or found objects. Students are encouraged to intentionally consider their art materials and how they represent their archetype. Students may choose to use one or both sides of the mask, make it functional (wearable), or create a stand for the mask. The following is the story of Maddie's archetype assignment, a radiation mask transformation, and the healing journey of her father John from a diagnosis of throat cancer. During their interview with Susan Ridley, both Maddie and John chose to use their real names to share their stories with others.

Radiation Masks

Head and neck cancers (HNC) are the seventh-most common type of cancer globally, accounting for approximately 660,000 new cases and 325,000 deaths annually (Sung et al., 2021). These cancers are often aggressive with high metastatic and recurrence rates (Basnayake et al., 2023). Depending on the type, location, and severity (stage) of the tumor, treatment may consist of a combination of surgery, radiation therapy coupled with chemotherapy, target therapy, and/or immunotherapy. Currently, almost 75% of HNC patients can benefit from radiation therapy during their cancer treatment (Alfouzan, 2021). Radiation therapy involves using high-energy radiation beams to target and destroy cancer cells in the affected area. During treatment, patients must use immobilization devices, such as custom-made masks or headrests, to ensure the patient remains in the same position throughout treatment. While lying down on the treatment table, these masks are placed over the patient's face, neck, and/or shoulders and secured to the treatment table to ensure minimal movement. These devices help precisely target the tumor and protect nearby healthy tissues. Individual radiation treatments may last up to 30 minutes, but some patients can undergo this treatment as frequently as daily for a number of weeks. One can imagine the psychological impacts of not only a cancer diagnosis but also essentially being bolted down on a table, immobilized daily for a number of weeks. Following a diagnosis, cancer patients might experience emotional distress (anxiety, depression, extreme fear), and frequently these patients experience loss of control, uncertainty, and a sense of powerlessness (Nainis et al., 2006).

Radiation masks may become a symbol of that experience, and the emotions associated with the treatment, though lifesaving, can also be quite traumatic. After radiation treatment is complete, patients keep the custom-made, mesh radiation masks. While it would be understandable for some patients to destroy or dispose of the masks, never to be seen again, there are some patients who have utilized the art process to transform these masks. It has been noted that some view the mask as a symbol of their torture, a perspective indicative of the experience of being immobilized on a treatment table. Some survivors may view the mask as a symbol representing self in a particular place and time. These individuals may view their masks as evidence of survival, strength, and overcoming adversity. Some patients have donated their masks to artists, to be transformed, and some choose to become the artist themselves. There are several art therapy programs dedicated to working with cancer patients, many located in oncology departments in hospitals or outpatient treatment centers. Art therapy can provide complementary psychosocial interventions to provide meaningful ways for patients to process the impact cancer has had on their lives and alleviate the distress caused by the diagnosis and intense treatment. The art making process gives the patient an opportunity to be in control, make choices, and reflect on one's experiences (Reiger et al., 2021). This arts-based transformative experience not only literally transforms the mask, but also offers an opportunity for the patient/artist to transform the experiences, creating new meaning in an adaptive way.

John's Journey

John was diagnosed with throat cancer in October 2019 and is now cancer-free. He was always positive and passionately believed that he would beat the disease and said, "I just knew it would be alright from the start" and that "this was not going to define me or end me."

Fitting for the Radiation Mask

One of the challenges of radiation for John was the suffocating feeling of being pinned into place unable to move while being bombarded with radiation to kill cancer cells. Each treatment took 15–30 minutes locked in place and one of his biggest fears was not being able to remain still, "and if you can't finish it, they have to start all over again." John remembered the fitting for the radiation mask:

So, they lay you down after you get the MRI machine running so they can see exactly where to place it and they heat this mask up and put it down over your face and it's really hot and wet. It goes over your face, and it instantly starts to constrict to pull on your face to fit every crack and crevice, so you are locked in when they use the radiation, it does not go where it is not supposed to go. That is the whole point of the mask. The mask puts you right where they want you so when they put the crosshairs of the radiation it stays there.

After-Effects of Cancer Treatment

For John, the mask was something that kept him alive, so he did not have any bad connotations towards it. He did not blame the mask; in fact, it helped him beat the cancer, "when something that scared you so much and it meant so many bad things that in the end it's not bad, it saved my life." It was the entire process that was difficult, and the feeling of being trapped unable to move during radiation that has stayed with him. For John, it was claustrophobic and traumatic, and the experience left a psychological mark. He said, "I was watching a movie with my son...about this guy getting in this tunnel and got to the end of the tunnel and it was narrow and a door at the end of it. He could not open the door, could not turn around to get out, and I had to leave the room, I just couldn't watch it, and that kind of stuff never bothered me before. It affected me quite a bit."

Maddie's Journey

Maddie chose to transform the radiation mask for the archetype project "because I wanted to turn something with such painful meaning into something beautiful and strong." She remembered her father calling it ugly and hoped that, once transformed, it would become a symbol of healing. Maddie chose the lover archetype because she sees it as a blessing and a curse. She said that she gets the most joy out of life by "making others feel happy even for a moment" and it is "something that I genuinely crave, to see a smile on someone's face just because of something I said and meant, is a beautiful thing." The lover archetype also represents her relationship with her father, because "we have been through a lot together and it made me think that no matter what we've been through together we will always love each other and that's why I chose it."

Outside Mask

Maddie decorated the outside of the mask with white and gold because it reminded her of her dad being a superhero, never getting sick, always there for her and her family, until faced with the real possibility that the cancer would get the better of him (Figure 21.1). "I did the white and gold to make it look almost futuristic with the eyelashes 'cause I thought they looked pretty, I wanted it to look pretty on the outside because we are very

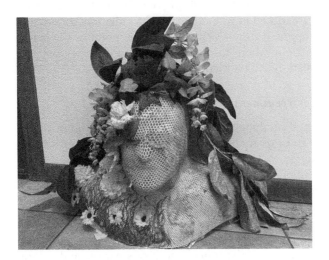

Figure 21.1 Outside of the radiation mask.

Photograph by Maddie Boyd.

strong, we are a loving family." Underneath the eye, there are blue splatters that represent tears, "when you fail to help someone, or fail to give them your all it hurts the Lover as well." Maddie believes "that with pain, we learn, and grow, and water grows flowers, quite like emotional sufferings can help push us towards self-growth."

Inside Mask

Maddie felt that the inside of the mask was her favorite part (Figure 21.2). She described it as "completely and messily covered in some burned, some ripped, some crumbled pieces of book pages ripped from one of my favorite childhood books because we were able to overcome the challenges we were facing." Maddie chose *Divergent, Harry Potter and the Order of the Phoenix,* and *Maximum Ride* because the main character was going through a huge self-realization and change for the better. Maddie said she loves Harry Potter, so tearing pages out of the book represented "a young me growing up a little bit." When she burned the edges of the pages, it wasn't done in a destructive way, but "showing that childhood image wasn't always real because it is not realistic." Maddie placed broken shards of mirrors on top of the pages "because we learned a lot about each other" and not "just the cancer but a lot of other things as well." For Maddie, "the glass is to show that no matter how lost in thought you are, you can still always look, and find yourself. Just how I have."

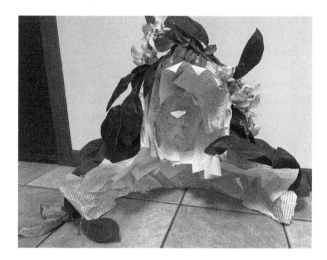

Figure 21.2 Inside of the radiation mask.
Photograph by Maddie Boyd.

Changing Relationships

Although John and Maddie's relationship has always been a close one; transforming the mask has brought them closer. The cancer treatment and challenges that family members went through have cemented their relationship and brought them closer still. John does not feel that the mask is ugly anymore. It helped his daughter to work through her emotions and deal with any lingering fears after his treatments. Maddie was excited to show her father the archetype mask and hoped he was proud of it. She really loved talking to him about the materials she chose and the meaning behind the mask. Transforming the radiation mask helped Maddie to talk about her feelings regarding her father's cancer treatments and fears for his health; it also reinforced her desire to be an art therapist:

I saw how it made me feel and how much it helped me get over that and heal from it. I always tell people how amazing art therapy is and I have always loved it, but that project really showed me what it can do. It was extremely healing for me and that is why I knew; I knew immediately that I wanted to keep going with it.

Giving Hope to Others

One of the reasons why Maddie entered her archetype mask in an exhibition of the work by students in the undergraduate creative arts therapy program was to give hope to others. She was very anxious because she didn't know how her father would feel with it being so public, but was excited because he was very open about his experiences. Maddie said, "It was wonderful, it was a very emotional night but a very good night." For John, the exhibition of the mask was an opportunity to help others. He said:

> I try to think of it as a positive now, try to tell everyone it's not going to define us, it's not the end, that it is an opportunity to help others. I'm always trying to find a way to be positive when I'm around other people. I don't like to carry negativity out there, there is enough of that, so maybe it's a good thing.

Conclusion

Including Jungian archetype masks as part of an undergraduate creative art therapy program can help students learn how art therapy can lend itself to self-discovery and process difficult experiences. Transforming radiation masks into works of art can help patients work through the negative psychological effects of their cancer treatment. John and Maddie share their experience and fears and how the therapeutic use of art transformed their relationship to each other and how they approach life.

References

Alfouzan, A. F. (2021). Radiation therapy in head and neck cancer. *Saudi Medical Journal, 42*(3), 247–254. https://doi.org/10.15537/smj.2021.42.3.20210660

Basnayake, B. W. M. T. J., Leo, P., Rao, S., Vasani, S., Kenny, L., Haass, N. K., & Punyadeera, C. (2023). Head and neck cancer patient-derived tumouroid cultures: Opportunities and challenges. *British Journal of Cancer, 128*(10), 1807–1818. https://doi.org/10.1038/s41416-023-02167-4

Jung, C. (1969). *The archetypes and the collective unconscious* (R. F. C. Hull, Trans.). Princeton University Press.

Nainis, N., Paice, J., Ratner, J., Wirth, J., Lai, J., & Schott, S. (2006). Relieving symptoms in cancer: Innovative use of art therapy. *Journal of Pain and Symptom Management, 31*(2), 162–169. https://doi.org/10.1016/j.panismypman.2005.07.006

Reiger, K., Lobchuk, M., Duff, M., Chernomas, W., Demczuk, L., Campbell-Enns, H., ... West, C. (2021). Mindfulness-based arts interventions for cancer care: A systemic review of the effects on wellbeing and fatigue. *Pscho-Oncology: Journals of the Psychological, Social and the Behavioral Dimensions of Cancer, 30*(2), 240–251. https://doi.org/10.1002/pon.5560

Sung, H., Ferlay, J., Siegel, R. L., Laversanne, M., Soerjomataram, I., Jemal, A., & Bray, F. (2021). Global cancer statistics 2020: GLOBOCAN estimates of incidence and mortality worldwide for 36 Cancers in 185 countries. *CA: A Cancer Journal for Clinicians, 71*(3), 209–249. https://doi.org/10.3322/caac.21660

Swan-Foster, N. (2018). *Jungian art therapy*, 1st ed. Taylor and Francis.

Chapter 22

The Avatar
Masks of Hope and Healing

Lucy Barbera

From time immemorial, masks have connected us to our culture, our ancestors, our original face, and our inner source of wisdom (Mizanoglu, 1998; Klein & Robison, 2003; King, 1979). The mask has given us and continues to provide us with a vital communication tool, a visual/tangible language to communicate emotions, feelings, and healing messages that words alone cannot communicate. The mask, as an expressive device, is not a new approach to healing trauma but an ancient practice. Examples are replete throughout myth, legend, and history, across culture, geographical areas, and time (Larsen, 1982; Campbell, 1949). Facilitating the use of the mask to assist clients in accessing their original face, their soul-teacher, to offer hope and healing during critical mental and medical health crises supports and strengthens the client when, understandably, they may be feeling powerless. The "mind-body" connection suggests that the condition of the physical body can impact one's psychological state and vice versa, with one's mental health impacting physical health.

Art Therapy and Cancer

The existential challenge that cancer poses has an enormous impact on a client's mental and physical health. Furthermore, Malchiodi (1999) wrote that "Art therapy is one of few therapies where the individual becomes actively involved in treatment through the process of art making and through the creation of a tangible product" (p. 16). Clients in physical or mental health crisis did not ask for their diagnosis, side-effects of treatment, nor their recurrences. Particularly with children, it is evident that they did not ask for treatments that leave them nauseous and in pain, necessitating lengthy hospitalizations, side effects, and relapses that require them to return to the hospital and miss significant instructional and social time due to required treatment protocols. Art making functions as a dynamic and effective healing tool because it gives clients full control at a challenging time where they understandably feel out of control. Art making

DOI: 10.4324/9781003365648-28

gives clients control of all decisions related to their expressive processes and products. In my research done over a one-year period in a children's hospital, clients were 75% more likely to choose mask making over a wide range of creative art therapy modalities offered, which makes this directive the preferred vehicle of control, expression, and healing. Consent forms were completed, and each client was given a pseudonym to guarantee anonymity.

Councill (1999) believes that returning the nexus of control to the client to facilitate their sense of agency is critical to their healing. She believed that "Crayons and paper cannot replace the powerful drugs of modern cancer treatment, but they can go a long way toward helping young people see themselves as active partners in the process of getting well" (p. 91). Is not the primary role of the therapist to provide a means of appropriate control to the client when they are feeling most vulnerable and powerless? Mask making supports clinicians and clients most effectively in its function as an empowerment tool, and guide.

The expressive use of masks as personal Avatars for hope and healing in the mental/medical health context will be examined through the following life-sustaining mask functions and case study indicators. This includes two images representing:

1. Mask as a vehicle of empowerment and transformation with an adult close to death with end stage cancer in private counseling.
2. Mask as Projector and Protector with two teens with virulent cancer diagnoses.
3. Mask as Concealer and Revealer with a teen in psychiatric crisis after a suicide attempt.

Masks as a Vehicle of Empowerment and Transformation

During a brief remission from cancer, Helene, a 65-year-old woman, was encouraged in therapy to focus her energy on creating a mask to support her healing. Her mask of "Hope" in Figure 22.1 (left) and her subsequent revision of her mask (right) demonstrate how the impact of her creative expression moved her to modify and rearrange the elements of her mask. Natalie Rogers (1993) urges clinicians to invite clients to use the expressive arts in tandem, what she termed the "creative connection," so they may explore their expression on deeper levels, opening other channels, if you will, to mine their expression for its gold. As a creative connection, Helene was invited to journal about her mask, which allowed her to glean insight and motivation for action that is evident in the following excerpt from her journal. In Helene's description of her mask making process, listen to her evocation of

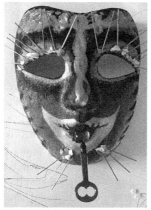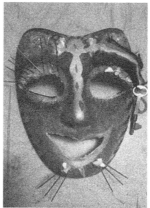

Figure 22.1 Helene's mask of "Hope" (left) and her mask transformed (right).
Photograph by the author.

several archetypes (universal symbols) including the key (golden symbol), the feminine (ancient feminine), and the eye (creative eye).

Observe how her trauma is represented and mitigated through the creative process:

> I found the journey into the mask to be a dynamic exploration into my psyche. The shape of the mask called forth a cat image that morphed into a golden symbol of the ancient feminine. The choice of nails represented the pain and loss I have had in my life. I revisited, briefly, some of the traumas, as I worked with it. I felt empowered by the creative process.

In her transformed mask, Helene decides to take her power back and remove the obstacle to her expression (her voice)!

> As I looked over the mask later, however, I realized that the mouth was shut by a key I chose to place there. Then I cut open the mouth and moved the key to a position submissive to the left feminine creative eye, bringing with it new lightness of expression.

Helene's mask functioned as Avatar, her teacher. It provided Helene with a means to personify, embody, and manifest: all functions of the archetype of the Avatar. Additionally, Helene's mask facilitated powerful realizations by identifying that her mouth (container for her voice) was locked, and with the sacred feminine as her ally, she was able to claim her power (through her expressive process and reflection) and unlock (open) her voice. The healing power of the mask's message is nothing less than the revelation of her Avatar, the quintessence of her highest wisdom.

Mask as Projector and Protector

In her seminal work on the origins of art, Dissanayake (1992a) says, "In order to include human history, human cultures, and human psychology, art must be viewed as an inherent universal (or biological) trait of the human species...." (p. 203). In her paleo-anthro-psycho-biological view of art "for life's sake," Dissanayake (1992b) encourages us to view art as an evolutionary product for survival. For the two children, whose masks are represented in Figure 22.2, survival is very much on their minds, as unbeknownst to them they drew on a very long tradition of art making as a survival mechanism. Both 13-year-old Ali and 14-year-old Heather were in hospital and being treated for virulent pediatric cancers.

Although these teens were in the same unit, they did not know nor interact with each other, as their stays in the hospital did not overlap. Remarkably, when asked to title or give their masks a voice, i.e. "What would your mask say, if it had a voice?", both had very similar titles. Ali titled his mask "He's Scared of Something" and Heather's mask's voice said, "It Scares Me." Notice that it is the mask who is "scared of something," not Ali. Also, notice "it scares me" regarding Heather's mask means the mask is scared, but Heather does not admit to being scared herself. In both instances, the mask revealed something that was difficult for each of them, as teenagers,

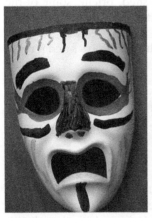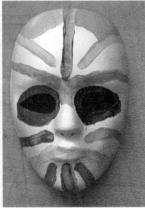

Figure 22.2 "He"s Scared of Something" (left) and Heather"s mask "It Scares Me." (right).
Photograph by the author.

to admit out loud: namely, their fear. For both, the mask served as foci for their projections, a safe place to express fear, far enough away from them not to be overwhelmed by it, a container to hold the undesirable emotion and keep it at a distance, and an object on which to release and project their fear. When they were overwhelmed with their physical illness and not able to take up precious psychological bandwidth, the mask served as their proxy.

Upon examination, both masks have other shared similarities. Even to the casual observer, they each can be seen as reminiscent of Japanese Kubuki masks. It has been noted that masks evolved "As objects of art, religion, or rituals...omnipresent in most of the world's cultures... The oldest Japanese vestiges date back to prehistory" (Japan Vibe, 2023). In the Kubuki tradition, masks are utilized ritualistically to express a variety of feelings, among them, fear, grief, anger, and despair. Not surprisingly then, when Ali was allowed to leave his room one evening, escorted by this art therapist, to show off his mask to the unit doctors and nurses, he chose instead to lurk around corners and pop out of closets and "scare" as many of them as possible in a very short span of time. After all the frightening procedures Ali had sustained, it was now his turn to frighten, and, ironically, the mask became not only the receptacle for his fear but his protector as well. His mask became his "power object" (Larsen, 1982) and necessary "ally" (Hillman, 1993). The doctors and nurses were very good sports during this spontaneous "healing ritual," and went out of their way, individually and collectively, to exaggerate their surprise and fear, delighting Ali and adding to the therapeutic value of the psychodrama.

Mask as Concealer and Revealer

Eva, a 17-year-old, was admitted to the children's hospital for medical stabilization after an attempted suicide. Evidence of repeated self-harming was apparent but still, the psychiatric nurse and social worker on the unit were having a very difficult time assessing Eva to determine the next steps for her treatment and, as her anxiety was so great, she became selectively mute. This is not rare in instances of trauma, and especially when self-inflicted. Although not able or willing to speak about her attempted suicide, Eva was eager to have this art therapist visit her and with that decision, she went from a passive state to an active one. Again, as Malchiodi (1999) observes "...art making requires that (children) become active participants in their health care."

The prospect of art making catalyzed Eva into action, and she created not one but two masks in rapid succession during the same session (Figure 22.3). She created the mask on the left first and titled it "Life & Death." Upon examination, this mask appeared congruent to Eva's situation. The mask is split down the middle vertically. The right side of the mask is completely

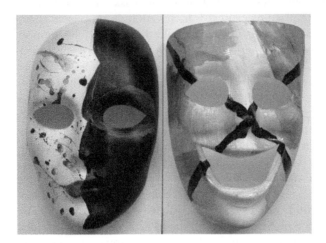

Figure 22.3 Eva's first mask, "Life & Death" (left), and Eva's second mask, "Truth-Teller" (right).

Photograph by the author.

black (death), and the left side of the mask is yellow with black splotches and red lips (life). One can imagine that if the "life" side of her mask is how she experiences her "life" then that life was fraught and chaotic. Researchers have identified "the need for control" as one of the primary motivations for self-harming behavior. Research also reveals that self-harming behavior increases the risk of suicide because it "normalizes" self-inflicted pain (Mitchell, 2021).

Eva's mask clearly shows how close her self-harming brought her to death. Was it carelessness during a routine habitual maladaptive behavior (cutting) or a deliberate attempt to end her life? This was still not entirely clear, not even to Eva, but the mask was a graphic, visual reminder of just how dangerously close her behavior brought her to death. When words are elusive, art making and, in particular, mask making allow the client to not only communicate with the therapist but just as importantly, allows communication with the self about the inner state of the self. Mask making provided a vehicle for expression for Eva to dialogue with herself, to question, to clarify, to be informed, to be heard. She looked at her mask (that may have had little meaning to the casual observer) and said, "That's exactly how I feel." The challenge in therapy is to find ways to help the client to see beyond and transform their pain, and so Eva was invited to imagine herself in the future, to imagine a time when she felt closer to her hopes and dreams.

Courageously, she chose a mask with a precut smile (the mask on the right). She painted the mask with care using many "bright" colors.

Kalsched (2013) posits that the mask "reveals more than it conceals." This is certainly true of Eva's second mask. After studying her mask for a few minutes, she abruptly and equally courageously picked up her brush, dipped it in black paint, and painted a black X across the brightly colored, smiling mask. Eva was able to express visually what realizing her hopes and dreams might feel like in the future, but the truth for her was that she was simply not there yet, thus the X. She titled her mask "Truth Teller." Her "inner wisdom child" seems to have been fully engaged during her mask making, and even the mask she created was unable to conceal Eva's true feelings: instead, the mask revealed them (Mizanoglu, 1998). During the art therapy session, Eva had appropriate "control" which was diametrically opposite to the "control" she sought in self-harming. Eva became more and more verbal, and bits and pieces of what precipitated her suicide attempt emerged. Her creative expression through the mask seemed to unlock her "voice." It was reported that later, in her session with the psychiatric nurse and social worker, the mask became a springboard and support for Eva to talk about what preceded and precipitated her hospitalization and provided the hospital staff with enough information to determine the best next steps for her treatment to optimize the possibility of her full healing and recovery.

Conclusion

The case studies presented in this chapter were selected to showcase the expressive use of the mask as a vital healing tool. The power of the expressive use of the mask for healing cannot be overstated. The mask, when utilized as an empowerment, transformation, projection, and protection tool, serves a critical healing function. The mask's ability to communicate with self and other, to reach and teach each client by providing a conduit between the unconscious and conscious to access innate wisdom, to embody the personal and transpersonal, to catalyze realization and action, and to coax the nonverbal to speak, is nothing short of miraculous. The Avatar mask is indisputably the interFACE of hope and healing.

References

Campbell, J. (1949). *The hero with a thousand faces*. Pantheon Books.
Councill, T. (1999). Art therapy with pediatric cancer patients. In C. Malchiodi (Ed.), *Medical art therapy with children* (pp. 75–93). Jessica Kingsley Publishers.
Dissanayake, E. (1992a). Art for life's sake. *Art Therapy: Journal of the American Art Therapy Association*, 9(4), 169–175. https://journals.sagepub.com/doi/full/10.1177/10778004211048379
Dissanayake, E. (1992b). *Homo aestheticus: Where art comes from and why*. University of Washington Press.

Hillman, J. (1993, November). *You can't fix it - And besides it ain't broke.* Keynote Address presented at the American Art Therapy Association 24th Annual Conference, Atlanta.

Japan Vibe. (2023). *Secrets and meaning of the Japanese masks.* https://japan-avenue.com/blogs/japan/japanese-mask.

Kalsched, D. (2013). *Trauma and the soul: A psycho-spiritual approach to human development and its interruption.* Routledge.

King, J. C. H. (1979). *Portrait masks: From the Northwest coast of America.* Thames and Hudson.

Klein, W., & Robison, B. (Eds.) (2003). *The other face: Experiencing the mask.* Bliss Plot Press.

Larsen, R. (1982). *Of masks and myths.* Association for Humanistic Psychology.

Malchiodi, C. (1999). Introduction to medical art therapy with children. In C. Malchiodi (Ed.), *Medical art therapy with children* (pp. 13–32). Jessica Kingsley Publishers.

Mitchell, M. (2021). *Self harm: Why teens do it and what parents can do to help.* Simon and Schuster.

Mizanoglu, M. (1998). *Persona: The Meaning behind the mask.* BGB Press, Inc.

Rogers, N. (1993). *The creative connection.* Science and Behavior Books.

Chapter 23

The Exploration of Using a Kintsugi-Inspired Mask Making Process in Addictive Behaviors

Charlene K. Michener

As a newly graduated art therapist, I wanted to explore the identities of addiction through masks that have been created, broken, and repaired with the Japanese technique, kintsugi. By exploring ceramic mask making, I hoped to gain insight into addiction and the perceived stigmas of my clients. All too often, the clients questioned "what is the point to continue fighting my addiction, when I've lost it all already?" During my first semester interning at an outpatient facility, I witnessed how support and being believed in could impact the chance of survival. It was the first winter during the 2019 COVID pandemic, and within my first week of being on-site, we had already lost two clients to overdose. Support from their counselors was not enough to help carry them through their hardships. The Centers for Disease Control and Prevention (CDC, 2020) stressed that with the state-regulated lockdown and stay-at-home orders, the population struggling with addictive behaviors was hit even harder than the general population. Individuals with addictive behaviors lost all human interactions and connections, meaning the biggest component to recovery, social engagement, and support was taken away (CDC, 2020). Once the lockdowns had been lifted and in-person engagements occurred, the rates of overdoses decreased drastically.

Ceramics and Kintsugi in Therapy

Ceramics are beneficial in a therapeutic setting for numerous reasons, including physicality of body expressions and mental processes for creating and observing the products (Sholt & Gavron, 2006). Ceramics promote transformative repair with the ability to parallel several factors of life, recovery, and therapeutic relations (Hinz, 2020; Keulemans, 2016; Nan et al., 2021; Wardi-Zonna, 2019), allowing unconscious materials to be amplified with personal meaning and symbols.

DOI: 10.4324/9781003365648-29

Expressive Therapies Continuum

It is important to understand how ceramics interact with the expressive therapies continuum (ETC) with regards to affect, kinesthetic, and sensory. The ETC is an art therapy tool that is used to describe the ways in which a client processes information during their interactions with art materials (Kagin & Lusebrink, 1978). Nan et al. (2021) demonstrated affect, or the emotional component of the ETC, by using clay in art therapy for emotional regulation. Czamanski-Cohen and Weihs (2016) found that combining body and mind engagements can increase acceptance and help to process emotions and explore self-identity. Nan (2021) found that sensory components such as touch, taste, smell, sound, and sight correlate to a natural cycle of life and how it relates to the individual using ceramics.

Kintsugi is based on the idea of taking what is broken and repairing it so that the once-damaged piece can be whole once more (Keulemans, 2016; Kumai, 2018; Santini, 2019). Kumai (2018) explained that "the practice of kintsugi is repairing broken vessels by sealing the cracks with lacquer and carefully dusting them with gold powder. The Japanese believe the golden cracks make the pieces even more precious and valuable" (p. 4). Kintsugi is also a metaphor for life, transforming one's damages, difficulties, or pain into a radiating gold light of beauty. Kumai suggested that each stage of the kintsugi process is not just a step of building, but each stage is a reflective process with deep purposes.

Addiction Masks

With my passion for helping individuals who struggle with addiction, I wanted to use a hands-on approach for them to identify their addiction. I hoped to not only provide insight into what their addiction looks like but to help clients realize that they have the power to break that addiction, repair the broken pieces, and accept the beauty of their past, present, and future self. While exploring the differences between addictive substances, I began by making a list of seven substances and paired them with seven types of clays: some were store-bought, homemade, or even sifted from the creek-bed outside. After finalizing my substance focuses and clays, I took roughly three weeks for each mask's creation and reflection process. The following are the steps for each stage (Figure 23.1):

1. Research substance of focus
2. Select clay medium type
3. Create mask
4. Let dry for a week
5. Add optional details such as paint or adhering objects on mask

6.   Break mask
7.   Repair with kintsugi
8.   Let it sit for a week
9.   Create final reflections

Each mask was handmade without the use of molds, which allowed for differences in size, shape, and density to occur. I kept a notebook for my writing processes before starting each mask. Then, when creating the final reflection for each mask, I'd lay the mask beside me and continue the writing process about the insight gained from the process. While reflecting on any connections to the substances and mediums, each mask provided a different insight into the addiction-identity. Reflection led to the possibility

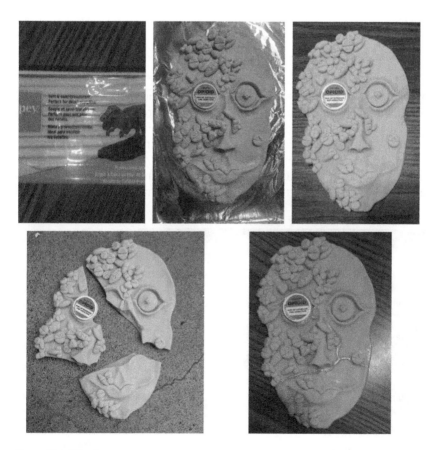

Figure 23.1 The Process.

Photograph by the author.

of understanding these individuals' choices and experiences: why, stigma, dysregulated emotions, "silent killer," thrive to fit in, side effects, and misunderstood.

A Counselor's Insights and Takeaways

Viewing these eight masks side by side as a series was thrilling (Figure 23.2). Looking at them left me with a breathtaking sensation and deep emotional response. These masks not only explored each individual addiction, but also provided insight to the addiction process. I was surprised that my journey through mask making provided such a better understanding of the world of addiction. I feel my masks have waited for the moment to allow their voices to be heard, much like those I have met on the streets waiting for an ear to listen. From this experience, I have found three main takeaways from the process.

Emotional Shutdown

When looking at my masks created to represent cocaine and methamphetamine addiction, I thought about how addiction causes an emotional shutdown. Whether the focus is on the stigma perceived by others or the internalized stigma of those who struggle with addictive behaviors, there are clearly outlined feelings of shame toward addiction (Birtel et al., 2017; Quinn, 2021). As mentioned by Birtel et al. (2017), the more shame and stigma imposed on an individual the more it will impact the recovery process. This was also supported by the US Department of Health and Human

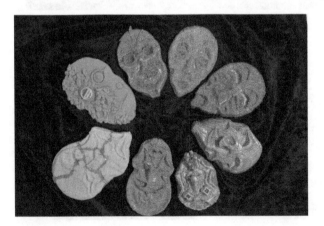

Figure 23.2 The Collection.
Photograph by the author.

Services (2019) when it emphasized the importance of understanding the value in support during the process to accept and connect to who they are and where supports currently lack.

From my professional experiences, emotions were among the top common struggles. Clients would easily verbalize feelings of shame for their addictions or be in denial about having addictive behaviors. Yet nearly all the clients I have worked with also struggled to express any emotion other than aggression. As the clients became more welcoming to the art therapy groups, there was a slow but gradual increase in expressing feelings and reconnecting to where the feelings of anger began to occur. What I also have observed is an overwhelming response from the clients when they engage with clay. There was a deeper investment with their art making time and when it came to sharing, they were able to hold a session with very limited input from me. They were able to express more feelings about the products they made and connect with each other over these emotions. Reflecting on insights gained through research and my mask making, it emphasizes how addictions and stigmas can manipulate and repress emotions. Yet through mask making and use of a ceramic medium, clients can understand their emotions and learn how to appropriately express them without aggression taking control.

The Great Misunderstanding

When looking at my masks created to represent the hallucinogens and heroin addiction, I thought about how addiction causes a large misunderstanding. The resistance to change in the stigma perceptions of the population appears to have resulted in a misunderstanding of these individuals struggling with addictive behaviors. Quinn (2021) addresses in her book how there are underlying reasons behind someone becoming addicted to substances, much more than the perceived "weakened character." As a result of this misunderstanding, these individuals express feeling as though they misunderstand themselves and their identity (Lang & Rosenberg, 2017). The first step in treatment is to focus on helping them face themselves and accept their past (Dunn-Snow & Joy-Smellie, 2011; Stephens et al., 2019). This often can be a long task for some, based on their self-values. Once this process has begun, the internal growth and transformative behaviors begin (Czamanski-Cohen & Weihs, 2016; Nan et al., 2021; Wardi-Zonna, 2019). Thanks to the focus on this, there will typically be a reduction in the past behaviors that led to relapse.

These individuals often shared their life stories about what led them to become addicted to their drug of choice and the community's responses that made them feel voiceless and misunderstood. One individual I worked with fit the definition of being misunderstood and afraid to grasp who he was as a person without his addiction. Many counselors at the site viewed this 19-year-old as a troublemaker who wasn't worth the struggle, for the fear of being physically or verbally attacked. Even his parents were intimidated and afraid of him. I saw what the other counselors claimed but I still never gave up on him. After a few weeks, we had a breakthrough where we understood through art. Through using metaphors, we could bypass his aggression and it was easier for him to communicate. By the end of his time at the facility, this individual transformed his past behaviors and could calmly take part in discussions about his after-care plans with no physical or verbal aggression. The client before discharge presented artwork he made to his family and identified it to them as where he was coming in, a ceramic creation of a dead tree in a graveyard with a noose around its branch (Figure 23.3). He then proceeded to snap that branch off the tree laying it on the ground by the trunk saying, "I no longer want to be dead; I want to survive." It represents that if we look beyond these stigma-perceived views on what addiction is, there could be a chance to help the individuals who are struggling find their journey to recovery.

From the Supports to the Risks

When looking at my masks created to represent the opioid and alcohol addictions, I was struck by how addiction can end in two very different

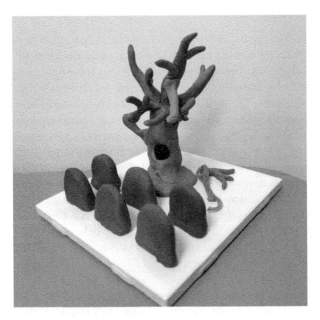

Figure 23.3 Cutting the Noose.
Photograph by the author.

ways: success or death. If changes could be made to improve the perceived outlook of individuals who suffer from addictive behaviors to support their desires to recover, death rates could begin to decrease. With the correct amount of support in helping these individuals understand themselves (Czamanski-Cohen & Weihs, 2016; Stephens et al., 2019) and how to express emotions once more, it could produce the required needs to support lasting change (Lang & Rosenberg, 2017; Nan, 2021). By creating a safe space without judgment through the process of art therapy, it could provide the effectiveness needed to initiate a change in the addiction taking control. When art therapy is combined with the Japanese kintsugi technique, a deeper life meaning can be implied to allow the clients to see the true beauty in honoring the past, even when it may not be defined as a good one (Keulemans, 2016; Kumai, 2018; Santini, 2019). Each of these individuals has a chance to understand the beauty within their broken pasts. However, if we continue to allow validation of stigma perceptions, there will only be more reports of overdoses (Centers for Disease Control and Prevention, 2020; National Institute on Drug Abuse, 2021). Possibly even more news reports showing how these individuals who lost their battle to substances are being covered up and misdocumented to numb the truth behind the losses (Gutman, 2021; Safai & Graber, 2020).

Client Process Observations and Reflections

During this process, I was able to really observe a difference in how everyone created their masks and how far they would commit to the process. There appeared to be a correlation between their processes and where they individually would land on the stages of change format. The stages of change are precontemplation, contemplation, preparation, action, and maintenance (Railhan & Cogburn, 2023). I found that clients in the group who identified with precontemplation, or as not being ready to admit they have an addictive behavior, often created positive or happy masks. While someone in the contemplation stage, or willing to accept their addictive behaviors are problematic but not prepared to make the needed changes, created a mask with more negative features but refused to break the mask they invested in. This aligned with hesitation and fears individuals may experience when trying to consider if it's time to give up their addictive behaviors and try to explore their recovery. For clients in the preparation stage, or willing to engage with the work required but needing support and guidance, they could break their masks with no problem. However, they also struggled to invest the time to find where the individual pieces belonged and repair the masks. Clients who were in the action or maintenance stage, implementing changes into their lives with little to no guidance, were able to repair their masks and often reflect on the correlations to how this mask was really a representation of not just their addictive identity but themselves.

Conclusion

Creating addiction masks using a ceramic medium that underwent a Japanese repair process called kintsugi helped me to understand the experiences of my clients. Some clients shared that they viewed their past addiction as a monster that would continually pull them backwards from success. Through mask making, breaking the pieces, and re-forming them, it helped to build self-acceptance and offered a new perspective, a sense of closure, and the empowerment to move forward. My observations also indicated a possible correlation between stages of change and the creation of their kintsugi mask. Further research is needed to support this hypothesis. However, my newly gained insight from the art making process has allowed me to better understand my clients and to help them build their golden repair for themselves.

References

Birtel, M. D., Wood, L., & Kempa, N. J. (2017). Stigma and social support in substance abuse: Implications for mental health and well-being. *Psychiatry Research*, 252. https://doi.org/10.1016/j.psychres.2017.01.097

Centers for Disease Control and Prevention. (2020, December 18). *Overdose deaths accelerating during COVID-19: Expanded prevention efforts needed*. Centers for Disease Control and Prevention. https://www.cdc.gov/media/releases/2020/p1218-overdose-deaths-covid-19.html

Czamanski-Cohen, J., & Weihs, K. L. (2016). The bodymind model: A platform for studying the mechanisms of change induced by art therapy. *The Arts in Psychotherapy*, 51, 63–71. https://doi.org/10.1016/j.aip.2016.08.006

Dunn-Snow, P., & Joy-Smellie, S. (2011). Teaching art therapy techniques: Mask-making, A case in point. *Art Therapy*, 17(2), 125–131. https://doi.org/10.1080/07421656.2000.10129512

Gutman, A. (2021, March 3). *Drug overdoses misreported as cardiac arrests, study shows*. MedShadow. https://medshadow.org/misreportedoverdoses/

Hinz, L. D. (2020). *Expressive therapies continuum: A framework for using art in therapy*. Routledge.

Kagin, S. L., & Lusebrink, V. B. (1978). The expressive therapies continuum. *Art Psychotherapy*, 5(4), 171–180. https://doi.org/10.1016/0090-9092(78)90031-5

Keulemans, G. (2016). The geo-cultural conditions of kintsugi. *The Journal of Modern Craft*, 9(1), 15–34. https://doi.org/10.1080/17496772.2016.1183946

Kumai, C. (2018). *Kintsugi wellness: The Japanese art of nourishing mind, body, and spirit*. HarperCollins.

Lang, B., & Rosenberg, H. (2017). Public perceptions of behavioral and substance addictions. *Psychology of Addictive Behaviors*, 31(1), 79–84. https://doi.org/10.1037/adb0000228

Nan, J. K. M. (2021). From clay to ceramic: An alchemical process of self-transformation. In L. Leone (Ed.), *Craft in art therapy: Diverse approaches to the transformative power of craft* (pp. 55–71). Routledge.

Nan, J. K. M., Hinz, L. D., & Lusebrink, V. B. (2021). Clay art therapy on emotion regulation: Research, theoretical underpinnings, and treatment mechanisms. *The Neuroscience of Depression*, 431–442. https://doi.org/10.1016/b978-0-12-817933-8.00009-8

National Institute on Drug Abuse (2021, July 1). *Breaking down the stigma of addiction: A witness' story through art.* National Institute on Drug Abuse. https://www.drugabuse.gov/videos/breaking-down-stigma-addiction-witness-story-throughart

Quinn, P. (2021). *Art therapy in the treatment of addiction and trauma.* Jessica Kingsley Publishers.

Railhan, N., & Cogburn, M. (2023, March 6). *Stages of change theory.* National Library of Medicine. https://www.ncbi.nlm.nih.gov/books/NBK556005/

Safai, Y., & Graber, M. (2020, February 27). The opioid crisis may be far worse than we thought, making the epidemic harder to fight. *ABC News.* Retrieved 2021, from https://abcnews.go.com/Health/opioid-crisis-worse-thought-making-epidemic-harderfight/story?id=69208304

Santini, C. (2019). *Kintsugi: Finding strength in imperfection.* Andrews McMeel Publishing.

Sholt, M., & Gavron, T. (2006). Therapeutic qualities of clay-work in art therapy and psychotherapy: A review. *Art Therapy, 23*(2), 66–72. https://doi.org/10.1080/07421656.2006.10129647

Stephens, M. B., Bader, K. S., Myers, K. R., Walker, M. S., & Varpio, L. (2019). Examining professional identity formation through the ancient art of mask-making. *Journal of General Internal Medicine, 34*(7), 1113–1115. https://doi.org/10.1007/s11606-019-04954-3

U.S. Department of Health and Human Services. (2019, June 20). *Health stigma and discrimination: A global, cross-cutting research approach.* National Institute of Mental Health. https://www.nimh.nih.gov/news/media/2019/health-stigma-and-discrimination-aglobal-cross-cutting-research-approach.

Wardi-Zonna, K. (2019). Finding Buddha in the clay studio: Lessons for art therapy. *Art Therapy, 37*(1), 42–45. https://doi.org/10.1080/07421656.2019.1656459

Chapter 24

Revealing ED

Therapeutic Uses of Masks in the Treatment of Eating Disorders

Lisa D. Hinz

The *DSM-5* diagnosis for eating disorders (ED; APA, 2013) ranges from caloric restriction and body wasting representative of anorexia nervosa (AN), to binge eating followed by self-induced vomiting in bulimia nervosa (BN) or no compensatory measures in binge eating disorder (BED). Individuals living with ED often suffer from physical, sexual, or emotional abuse and exhibit difficulties with emotion regulation (Feinson & Hornik-Lurie, 2016; Ketisch et al., 2014). They demonstrate high levels of cognitive rigidity and have been characterized as perfectionistic and overcontrolled (Isaksson et al., 2021; Schilder et al., 2021). At the same time, an undercontrolled, moderately impulsive, and behaviorally and emotionally dysregulated personality type has also has been noted (Isaksson et al., 2021). Those who develop ED have been characterized as extremely caring individuals who often have been called upon (explicitly or implicitly) to care for parents with addictions or debilitating mental or physical illnesses (Hinz, 2006). This pattern of early caretaking teaches young people to deny their own thoughts, feelings, and needs, and perhaps to develop a pleasing persona to interact with an adult world not completely comprehensible to them. ED frequently begins during adolescence when body image concerns are at the forefront of developmental issues; body image dissatisfaction has been shown to be a prospective risk factor for the development of ED (Prnjak et al., 2021). Hunter (2012) has posited that ED represents one way of dealing with the tremendous body image changes that occur during adolescence and that art therapy is uniquely positioned to aid in exploring and changing body image dissatisfaction. ED is notoriously difficult to treat, characterized by high rates of relapse and with only half of those treated remaining symptom-free (Delinsky et al., 2010).

Art Therapy and the Use of Masks in Eating Disorders

Art therapy can be particularly helpful in the treatment of ED due to its ability to circumvent language, especially the tendency to engage in the

DOI: 10.4324/9781003365648-30

excessive rationalization and intellectualization so often encountered in AN (Hinz, 2006). A recent review of the use of art and music therapy in the treatment of ED indicated that art therapy may be effective at reducing negative emotional states in the treatment of ED (Pedra Cruz Bettin et al., 2023). The authors noted the importance of reducing negative affect in the treatment of ED because negative affect often triggers binge eating in BN and caloric restriction in AN.

The use of masks in art therapy can be helpful in reducing the tension associated with opposing mind states and emotions, which could make it effective in the treatment of ED (Haeyen et al., 2022). Mask making and the process of interacting with masks can be challenging (Hinz & Ragsdell, 1990; Janzing, 1998; Lay, 2021). The use of masks in art therapy is an emotionally evocative and powerful intervention that does not always lead to a beneficial outcome. Fear of the mask should be respected because it is likely related to a fear of loss of identity or loss of self (Janzing, 1998). The mask is viewed as a mediator between the everyday self and the dramatized self with infinite possibilities existing due to the presence of the mask/mediator (Landy, 1985). Putting on a mask closes the distance between the mundane self and the desired self and thus has tremendous therapeutic potential when cautiously observed and implemented (Landy, 1984).

Emotional Expression and Emotional Regulation

When carefully monitored, masks can be used in the treatment of individuals with ED to encourage or augment emotional expression as one form of emotion regulation (Feinson & Hornik-Lurie, 2016; Isakson et al., 2021). When the face is masked, a disinhibitory effect occurs, characterized by increased willingness to experiment with new behaviors and attitudes (Janzing, 1998). This disinhibitory effect is perhaps related to the use of the face to effortfully conceal feelings (Turner, 1981). Therefore, when the face is masked, authentic emotions can be disclosed. This revelatory effect can be particularly powerful in the treatment of ED, where perfectionism and the denial of emotions, feelings, and needs often has silenced the individual. Clients with ED demonstrate more maladaptive than adaptive emotion regulation strategies, especially regarding anger and sadness. Some of the first masks created in art therapy can be used to describe the current level of emotional expression. Using the face form has been described as increasing the emotional attachment to the work and making it more personal and emotionally evocative (Landy, 1984, 1985).

The mask in Figure 24.1 was created by Amber, a 17-year-old Caucasian woman suffering from BN who used it to demonstrate that she never felt free to express her thoughts and feelings in her family of origin. She understood from family dynamics that she was meant to enhance the family image

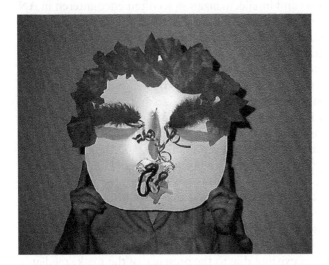

Figure 24.1 Amber's mask revealing that purging through self-induced vomiting was a way to have a voice in her family.

Photograph by the author.

by being perfect. She never complained about the academic, athletic, and social responsibilities placed upon her by her alcoholic father and her silent, complicit mother; she complied. However, after creating and interacting with her first mask, Amber stated that she realized that purging was a way for her to voice her rage at her demanding parents.

In order to learn and embrace greater emotional expression, clients can be encouraged to create masks exemplifying different emotional expressions such as anger, anxiety, and sadness and then to use the masks to experiment with the universal expression of these diverse emotions. After some practice, and when this general emotional expression is effectively in place, individuals can create different masks expressive of their own personal emotions and use them to specifically address emotionally charged issues in their lives, such as the belief that to be loved they must be perfect.

Integration of Opposites

Another way to confront perfectionism is to create an "inside-outside" mask in which the outside of the mask portrays the acceptable, if not perfect, persona that the client presents to the world. The inside of the mask is created to represent the hidden aspects of the self (Kruczek, 2001). This type of mask serves as a mediator between the conscious and the unconscious; between the authentic self and the aspects of the personality deemed more suitable to present publicly (Landy, 1985). When carefully managed, a dialogue can occur between opposing parts of the personality and this encounter can be an invitation for their successful integration (Haeyen et al., 2022). This type of externalized inner dialogue can be powerful for those who have been unable to communicate their thoughts, feelings, or needs directly or for those who typically engage in excessive rationalization or stereotypical communication.

Examining Stereotypical Presentations

Stereotypical presentations (or projections) can be addressed directly by using masks to represent them. Hinz (2006) discussed the use of masks to represent positive or negative stereotypes or projections by having clients with ED create a list of characteristics of three persons they greatly dislike. These traits were then used as the foundation of a mask to illustrate a stereotypical figure, and were further mined as prompts to more deeply examine the qualities represented. Typically, after interacting with the negative mask, ED clients are prone to claim all the negative qualities in a self-condemning fashion. Clients can interact with the mask again to determine its positive qualities or benefits. For example, a mask that typifies a "selfish" person perhaps can be seen as one who is not so much self-centered as one who engages in appropriate self-care.

Subsequently, Hinz (2006) had clients create a list of three people whom they deeply admire, a corresponding list of highly regarded qualities, and a positive mask. In their later interactions with the new mask, clients can be gently encouraged to investigate how they possess these favorable traits and how they are demonstrated in their behavior. According to Hinz (2006), it is often more difficult for ED clients to embrace their positive qualities than the negative ones. However, speaking of themselves from the masks can set the stage for effective internalization of the highly regarded qualities.

Imposter Syndrome and Shame Reduction

As was mentioned earlier, many people who develop ED have acted as childhood caretakers of physically or mentally ill parents. Young women who develop ED are likely to have witnessed parental conflicts, arguments, and domestic violence. In one study, ED women reported that they were expected as children to care for their abused mothers while absorbing emotional abuse from them (Ketisch et al., 2014). The mask in Figure 24.2 was created by Clara, a 20-year-old Latinx female with BN who was a caretaker of her mother and younger brother after her physically abusive father left the family when she was 11 years old. Clara already had functioned as a translator for both parents in the school system and at family members' medical appointments. After her father left and her mother went to work

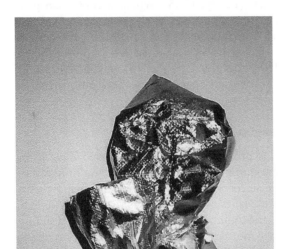

Figure 24.2 Clara's mask for her mask exemplifying the imposter syndrome and her feelings of shame.

Photograph by the author.

outside the home, Clara grocery shopped, cooked meals for the family, and cleaned the house because her mother was too tired and sad to do so. Clara was never taught the skills required of her to act as her mother's translator, protector, and caretaker, but she pretended to know it all and she felt constantly judged by others as she navigated the dominant culture that she did not fully understand.

Clara explained that the mask showed a fearful child disguised as an adult – she made a mask for her mask! Clara said that she was embarrassed to admit that she did not know what she was doing as she made her way in the adult world. Clara further explained that she used a reflective material to create the masks so that people would not be able to look intensely at her; instead, their own critical reflections would be shown to them. Despite her self-doubt and the many demands on her at home, Clara achieved top marks in school and was enrolled in a program to help her succeed at university.

However, regardless of her success, the young woman still viewed herself as a child posing as an adult. Creating, making meaning of, and interacting with the mask helped Clara understand the roots of her self-doubt and shame, develop empathy for the child inside, and embrace her successful young adult self.

Archetypal Figures

An encounter with a childlike figure through mask making can bring up the topic of archetypal figures that represent unconscious content shared among all human beings. Although archetypal work is not often pursued with adolescent clients, creating masks to represent the patterns and flow of our shared humanity can be engaging with adolescent clients (Martin, 2018). They can be encouraged through guided visualization to understand and connect with the various child archetypes. An examination of the past through the lens of universal archetypes often can moderate personal suffering, nurture self-compassion, and, if done in a group, increase connection. Connections made with the trickster or the hero archetype can suggest novel ways of interacting in the world and help individuals embrace new strengths. Active practice while wearing the archetypal mask can foster new attitudes, ways of communicating, and types of action. Because the archetypal connection is universal and part of common humanity, the exploration often takes on a theatrical tone that allows for greater expansion and exploration of the newfound attitudes, communication patterns, and behaviors.

Body Image

Masks can be used to address body image issues, societal pressures to meet Eurocentric beauty standards, and the disconnection between mind and body often experienced by those with ED (Hunter, 2012). Wearing a mask focuses attention on breathing in a positive way that can increase the connection between body and mind (Janzing, 1998). This attention to breathing can be a first step in reestablishing trust in the physical body that many individuals with ED feel betrayed them. Masks can be made to delineate, question, protest, and reject impossible body image standards. Due to the disinhibitory effect of wearing a mask, clients reported that they have questioned norms and made statements that they never had before.

When the face is covered with a neutral mask, self-consciousness is raised about what is occurring in other parts of the body (Turner, 1981). Thus, a neutral, ready-made mask form can be used to cover the face when the therapist wants to highlight feelings and movements in the rest of the body. Using the neutral mask, ED clients can recognize how much of their emotional lives occur in their head and how little in their body. The split between the mind and body, and helping ED clients reconnect with the wisdom of their bodies, is a central theme in ED treatment (Hinz, 2006).

Identity Formation

The fundamental task of adolescence is identity formation and to that end, it is paramount that persons with ED be able to separate themselves from the disorder (Hinz, 2006). Frequently, identification with the disorder is so strong that the client refers to themself as being "an anorexic" or "a compulsive eater." Often the initial action in treatment, and an effective use of art therapy, is to separate the person from the disorder. The mask in Figure 24.3 was created by Celia, a 16-year-old Chinese American female who struggled to separate herself from AN, which had defined her for three

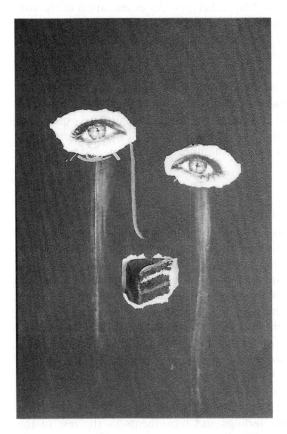

Figure 24.3 Celia's mask demonstrates her initial identification with her eating disorder.
Photograph by the author.

years. However, the mask allowed her to concretely view this dangerous association and was a first step towards disentangling herself from it. After interacting with her mask, Celia was less prone to say, "I am anorexic" and more likely to say, "I am Celia and I am in treatment for anorexia nervosa."

Stephens et al. (2019) described a three-mask method to explore identity transformation in medical students from the start to the end of their medical school training. The same process can be used to examine the transformation of identifying ED treatment. The first mask is created at the outset of treatment and explores the question, "who am I?" and asks the creator to ponder what they present to others. This first mask can examine and display issues such as: where I am from, what I like, what my hopes/fears and likes/dislikes are. The second mask, made midway through treatment, is illustrative of the question, "who have I become?" This mask can be accompanied by a guided visualization that requires the ED client to remember who they were when they started treatment and to develop an image of who they are now. Finally, the last mask addresses the question, "who do I want to be?" A guided meditation would include an exploration into what they want to say about their experience as they transition out of treatment, what elements of the person remained the same, what changed, and what is hoped for in the future.

The three masks below (Figure 24.4) were created by Lilia, a 14-year-old Latinx girl undergoing intensive outpatient treatment for AN, which included both individual and group art therapy. When she entered treatment, Lilia created the "who am I" mask. As can be seen in the image, it is relatively plain and lacking in personal detail. Lilia explained that she created the mask to portray her need to be perfect, agreeable, and happy all the

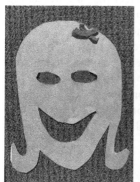 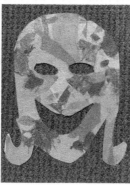 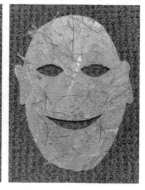

Figure 24.4 Lilia's three masks: "who am I?" (left), "who have I become?" (middle), and "who I want to be" (right).

Photograph by the author.

time. She said that she felt in her family of origin that she was not supposed to stand out or call attention to herself for any reason. Ironically, the AN caused her to become the center of attention: first, among her friends who wanted to know her secret to successfully losing weight; second, among her family who were worried that she might be ill; and last, among the school personnel who insisted that she get medical attention after she fainted at school. When asked to introduce herself from her mask, Lilia was reticent. When she did talk, Lilia spoke in a voice that was barely audible. She stated that she was "nothing special" and she could not identify one quality that made her different from others. As treatment continued, Lilia disclosed that she was raped by an older male cousin when she was eight years old; she had never before disclosed the sexual abuse.

Lilia's second mask was created about four weeks into an eight-week treatment program. At that time, she repurposed her first mask to answer the question, "who have I become?" Lilia explained that she was "all over the place" and feeling emotions that she thought were evident "all over my face." She said that during treatment she learned that the ED developed when her body began to develop at adolescence. She realized that she had wanted to shrink from male notice. Lilia also explained that her previous preoccupation with weight, caloric restriction, exercise, and food restriction, warded off feelings. In treatment, she began to experience her emotions and at times felt overwhelmed by them, which she portrayed in the mask. Lilia's other work in art therapy helped her address sexual abuse, body image concerns, learn new emotion regulation strategies and assertiveness skills, and prepared her for life after the treatment program.

The final mask represented "who I want to be" and her response was "put together, natural, and confident." She explained that put together meant calm, and natural meant that she would not feel that she was acting falsely as she had prior to treatment. Lilia claimed that she had not given her other masks names because she did not feel attached to them. This mask, however, she named ED. Lilia explained that she could now intentionally take on the characteristics that she felt her mask embodied: a strong persona which she thought of as quietly powerful, somewhat masculine, and protective. Although she admitted that she had a long way to go, at the end of her treatment Lilia saw herself as more capable of taking care of herself – through verbal, intellectual, emotional, and physical means – and these were skills that she wanted to continue to develop.

Conclusion

Eating disorders are increasing across the world and these difficult-to-treat disorders require innovative interventions. This chapter highlighted the many ways that art therapists can employ masks in the treatment of ED. Due to the disinhibitory effects of wearing a mask, the experience can be quite emotionally charged and should be carefully monitored. Used with caution, making and interacting with masks can aid in emotional expression and emotion regulation, foster the integration of opposite feelings or opposing parts of the personality, and facilitate the examination of stereotypical presentations of the self. Using masks can introduce archetypal figures and their unique strengths, challenge body image concerns, and aid in identity formation. The case illustrations provided examples of how masks were individually interpreted and successfully employed in the treatment of ED.

References

American Psychiatric Association. (2013). *Diagnostic and statistical manual of mental disorders*, 5th ed. Author.

Delinsky, S. S., St. Germain, S. A., Thomas, J. J., Craigen, K. E., Fagley, W. H., Weigel, J. J., ... Becker, A. E. (2010). Naturalistic study of course, effectiveness, and predictors of outcome among female adolescents in residential treatment for eating disorders. *Eating and Weight Disorders*, 15(3), e127–e135. https://doi.org/10.1007/BF03325292

Feinson, M. C., & Hornik-Lurie, T. (2016). Binge eating & childhood emotional abuse: The mediating role of anger. *Appetite*, 105, 487–493. https://doi.org/10.1016/j.appet.2016.05.018

Haeyen, S., Ziskoven, J., Heijman, J., & Joosten, E. (2022). Dealing with opposites as a mechanism of change in art therapy in personality disorders: A mixed methods study. *Frontiers in Psychology*, 13, 1–15. https://doi.org/10.3389/fpsyg.2022.1025773

Hinz, L. D. (2006). *Drawing from within: Using art in the treatment of eating disorders*. Jessica Kingsley Publishers.

Hinz, L. D., & Ragsdell, V. (1990). Using masks and video in group psychotherapy with bulimics. *The Arts in Psychotherapy*, 17(3), 259–261. https://doi.org/10.1016/0197-4556(90)90009-F

Hunter, M. R. (2012). *Reflections of body image in art therapy: Exploring self through metaphor and multimedia*. Jessica Kingsley Publishers.

Isaksson, M., Ghaderi, A., Wolf-Arehult, M., & Ramklint, M. (2021). Overcontrolled, undercontrolled, and resilient personality styles among patients with eating disorders. *Journal of Eating Disorders*, 9(1). https://doi.org/10.1186/s40337-021-00400-0

Janzing, H. (1998). The use of the mask in psychotherapy. *The Arts in Psychotherapy*, 25(3), 151–157. https://doi.org/10.1016/S0197-4556(98)00012-4

Ketisch, T., Jones, R., Mirsalimi, H., Casey, R., & Milton, T. (2014). Boundary disturbances and eating disorder symptoms. *American Journal of Family Therapy*, 42(5), 438–451. https://doi.org/10.1080/01926187.2014.912103

Kruczek, T. A. (2001). Inside-outside masks. In H. G. Kaduson & C. E. Schaefer (Eds.), *101 more favorite play therapy techniques* (pp. 70–74). Jason Aronson.

Landy, R. (1985). The image of the mask: Implications for theatre and therapy. *Journal of Mental Imagery*, 9(4), 43–56. https://www.researchgate.net/publication/232419248

Landy, R. J. (1984). Puppets, dolls, objects, masks, and make-up. *Journal of Mental Imagery*, 8(1), 79–89. https://www.researchgate.net/publication/232479296

Lay, R. P. M. H. (2021). Portrait masks, appropriated space, and an overseas art experiential: Nature as critical catalyst in the practice and training of art therapy. *Creative Arts in Education and Therapy*, *7*(1), 59–70. https://doi.org/10.15212/CAET/2021/7/6

Martin, E. M. H. (2018). *A theoretical inquiry exploring archetypal art therapy with adolescent clientele* [Unpublished Master's Thesis]. Concordia University.

Pedra Cruz Bettin, B., Urquiza Nogueira, L., Bertasso de Araujo, P. A., & Antunes, L. C. (2023). Visual art- and music-based interventions as adjuvants in the treatment of eating disorders: A systematic review and a theoretical model. *Arts & Health: An International Journal for Research, Policy and Practice*. https://doi.org/10.1080/17533015.2023.2218408

Prnjak, K., Hay, P., Mond, J., Bussey, K., Trompeter, N., Lonergan, A., & Mitchison, D. (2021). The distinct role of body image aspects in predicting eating disorder onset in adolescents after one year. *Journal of Abnormal Psychology*, *130*(3), 236–247. https://doi.org/10.1037/abn0000537.supp

Schilder, C. M. T., Sternheim, L. C., Aarts, E., van Elburg, A. A., & Danner, U. N. (2021). Relationships between educational achievement, intelligence, and perfectionism in adolescents with eating disorders. *International Journal of Eating Disorders*, *54*(5), 794–801. https://doi.org/10.1002/eat.23482

Stephens, M. B., Bader, K. S., Myers, K. R., Walker, M. S., & Varpio, L. (2019). Examining professional identity formation through the ancient art of mask-making. *JGIM: Journal of General Internal Medicine*, *34*(7), 1113–1115. https://doi:org/10.1007/s11606-019-04954-3

Turner, C. (1981). Body image stress in neutral mask work. *The Arts in Psychotherapy*, *8*(1), 37–41. https://doi.org/10.1016/0197-4556(81)90017-4

Part VI

Celebrating Life Stories

Chapter 25

Mask as a Starting Point
Usability in Crisis Sand Therapy

Natallia Sakovich

The persona archetype is often associated with the mask that one wears in different social roles to conform to expectations imposed by others. The mask can hide our true self from the world and our shadow becomes the vessel for all the things that we dislike about ourselves (Jung, 1981). This disconnect between our inner thoughts and feelings and our outward actions can result in an emotional breakdown and a crisis of identity where the inner and outer worlds clash (Adler & Hull, 1971). The persona can deprive an individual of opportunities to express their true emotions and the shadow becomes Pandora's box, where individuals keep their strongest destructive states. Only the mask of death can stop the pain.

Sand Therapy

Sand therapy helps us to explore our inner Pandora's box and to recognize masks that may ruin our lives. This is a process in which the therapist provides the client with a tray or box filled with sand and the choice of a variety of miniature figurines to create a play world within a safe confined space. Ruth Ammann (1991) called the sand tray a soul garden, a space for the expression of the client's inner world. The therapist facilitates the processing of this inner world and creates a protected field where the client can let masks out and allow the inner voice to speak. Sand therapy opens a pathway to the client's emotional core. The client features images existing in their inner and outer world, allowing them to disclose their inner true self and making the unconscious visible.

Dora Kalff (2003) developed sandplay therapy after learning the world technique from Margaret Lowenfeld, a British pediatrician and child psychologist and one of the founders of art therapy. Kalff developed the technique in the late 1950s by combining several techniques from her Jungian training and Eastern philosophy. She based her method on "the creation of free and protected space" where any client (an adult or a child) was able to express and explore their inner world, transforming their experience and

DOI: 10.4324/9781003365648-32

emotions into three-dimensional images of the emotional state. In this way, conflicts are transferred from the inner to the outer world through symbolic objects placed in sand. Unconscious processes become visible and therefore acknowledged and processed.

Masks and Sandplay Therapy

I believe that the set of symbolic objects used in sandplay therapy should include masks reflecting various emotional states such as crisis, pain, and loss. Such symbols used in sand pictures help clients enter the shadow concealed by the mask, to face the shadow in the safe psychotherapeutic environment in order to integrate it and to overcome the crisis. The set of masks used in sandplay therapy becomes an entry to the shadow field, the dark side of inner conflicts, allowing the client to visualize them and make them concrete. These are the masks of emotions and states, masks reflecting madness and naivety, masks for different social roles and genders, the masks of ego states, and the masks of major archetypes. Clients can also make a mask using modeling clay in a sandbox or mixing sand and water to create figurines. Modeling sand is also good for shaping due to its high plasticity.

Anna's Story

Surviving infidelity is the headline of the story. My client (let's call her Anna) was a young 35-year-old woman at the time of the sandplay therapy treatment. She had been married for 14 years and had a ten-year-old son when she discovered her husband's infidelity. When Anna turned to me for help, I noticed that she was overwhelmed with emotions. I thought that sandplay would help Anna to release trapped emotions, especially her grief of betrayal. We agreed on ten one-hour weekly sessions. All sessions started with reflections on the week, and then Anna got to work. A typical task was to set up a world, whatever she wanted it to be, using figurines and sand. During the construction, I was by her side observing and taking notes in silence. When the sand painting was completed, we made a journey into Anna's world. I asked her to tell me in detail about what she had built and the figurines she had chosen. Then I asked follow-up questions based on what Anna had said and on the archetypal and symbolic meanings of figurines, linking them to her lived experience. We reflected on it at the end of each session. It was important to analyze the secrets that Anna's mind had shared with us.

Anna felt devastated by the trauma of betrayal and her sand pictures were overwhelmed with pain and despair. The first figurines were created without miniatures, by hand only. Emerging images evoke many feelings and become a bridge to understanding the client's emotions. I felt anxious watching Anna's nervous fingers creating sand ripples. It was like lake-surface ripples caused by the wind blowing before the hurricane. She called her first figurine "The Mask" (Figure 25.1). It resembles a cosmetic or masquerade face mask with two holes for eyes and a woven-look top structure with the client's fingerprints. Staring at this image, she reflected on how she could have missed what was happening. Brushing sand from eye holes, Anna asked herself:

> How did I fail to notice it? He would go into another room and kept texting someone. He was not kind to me and hardly ever called our son to play football. He was no longer with us, and I was blind. I thought he worked hard and was tired, and I would better leave him alone.

The mask itself is very reminiscent of the image of an owl famous for the power of wide vision. In Anna's monologue, we see that she is like an owl looking around to see from different angles what has happened to her and her husband and to accept it.

During the second session, Anna picked the mask of sorrow (Figure 25.2a) from the selection of miniatures on the shelves and started talking about her grief. She didn't want to work with sand like she did at the first session and didn't want to take other figurines. Anna said:

> I spotted this mask at the first session. It's me crying! I'm crying because when he left, I lost a part of my life, as if I was deprived of everything we had. As if I lost my son. I would never have a baby from this marriage. My son would never have a brother he had dreamt of.

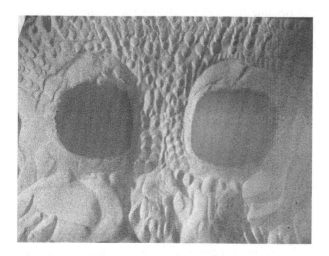

Figure 25.1 The Mask.

Photograph by the author.

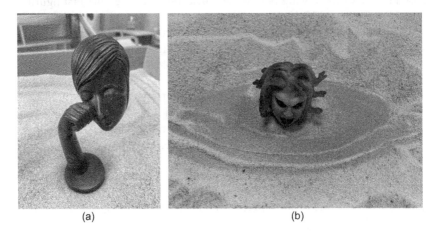

(a)   (b)

Figure 25.2 The Mask of Sorrow and the Mask of Anger.

Photograph by the author.

The husband decided to leave the family and filed for divorce. The sadness gripped her. She was eager to save their marriage, but he refused. Looking at the mask of sorrow and touching it now and then, Anna talked about how they had been classmates at school, how they had moved to another city and started building a family, how their son had been born and how they had made plans for the future. The mask of sorrow helped to release emotions with tears and became the wailer assisting the young woman in coping with her loss. In the end of the session, Anna thanked the wailer (the mask of sorrow) for sharing her grief and for visualizing it. Anna's environment, her friends and family encouraged her not to be sad or grieve because divorce was a normal thing. During the session, Anna put on the mask of sorrow that helped process loss.

The mask of the Gorgon Medusa was to appear at the next session (Figure 25.2b). The client gave her figurine the title of "the anger." First, she cleared the space of the sand tray with her hands to form an eye-shaped lake with the Gorgon Medusa in the center. Anna felt angry at her husband, who had betrayed her and their child; at her parents-in-law, who had supported their son; at their common friends who had "liked" the photos of her husband and his mistress when they were still married, etc. Looking at the Gorgon Medusa, we recalled Medusa's story – the story of betrayal and the spell. Anna had a strong desire to turn everyone around to stone, even her son, who reminded her of her husband. This mask facilitated the validation of aggression and anger as the Medusa-pupil became overwhelmed with anger towards the cheater and the whole world. The mask of Medusa became the lens refracting the betrayal trauma.

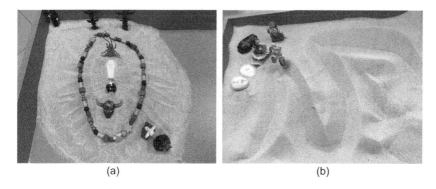

(a)   (b)

Figure 25.3 The Meeting and the Grave.

Photograph by the author.

At the following session, Anna kept stirring the sand with her hands to create hills and slides and finally built up a figurine named "the meeting" (Figure 25.3a). The miniature of a girl in a dress featured the client, and opposite was her husband represented by a beautiful prince holding a rose in his hand and asking a girl to dance. We see a perfect image of a couple: a beautiful prince and a beautiful girl. She told me that she had had a dream where they were talking as if nothing had happened. Using figurines, Anna said "I dreamed that we were standing outside our house, there was a bench and nice bushes, and we were talking and laughing like we used to do. Like nothing had happened. I miss that time so much." At the same time, Anna placed a coffin in the shadow of the girl and two masks next to it, the mask of cry and the mask of death. The enchanted clock from Disney's *Beauty and the Beast* (1991) is on the other side.

Looking at the scene she created, Anna reflected on how she would like to talk to her husband, to make him apologize, to make him understand what he had done to their family. Speaking about the coffin behind her figure, she suggested that it was time to bury this relationship and to say goodbye to it. Although she made all efforts "to be strong" for her parents and son, signs of depression became visible. Anna said that she could not sleep, she had no appetite, and did not feel like doing anything at all, as if all her energy had run out. Even her son was annoying because he needed her help and care. Two masks lying next to each other represent two alternating roles: a woman crying over her loss and a frozen woman with a dead emotional state. Anna felt that her personal clock had been temporarily enchanted; time runs differently in this crisis period.

At the next meeting, Anna built the grave in the sand tray (Figure 25.3b). The client carefully gathered all sand in the tray to make a hill with a grave on top. She decorated the grave with handmade wooden beads and placed two totem poles. She selected the mask of a demon. At the very last moment, she accommodated the miniature of an elderly man in the upper left corner, along with two Harry Potter characters: Snowy Owl and Hagrid with a dragon egg in his hands.

Anna talked about her husband's infidelity and the loss of marriage as death. In this grave, she buried her hopes including those to have a second child from this marriage, her expectations, and illusions. She was scared because she did not wish to bury her past and herself in the relationship. The elderly man was watching or safeguarding the grave. This is the father's miniature supporting the client in her trauma survival. The mask of the demon can indicate signs of the demonization of the husband who betrayed Anna and left the family. Also, it reflects her shadow, demonstrating her madness of grief, her anger, rage, and aggression. Hagrid seems to duplicate an animistic perspective and the father's image. Being a gamekeeper in J.K. Rowling's books (1997), Hagrid had access to the most terrifying and scary things in Hogwarts. Choosing this figure revealed the client's ability to tame her dragons and other shadow content, and to stay in contact with them without killing or denying.

The mask of reflection appears in the center of the sand tray in the next figurine. "Reflection" was the title that Anna gave to her figurine. The mask divides the figurine into two parts. Anna reflected on her roles in marriage before it happened, thinking about what kind of bride, friend, wife, and mother she was. The wise men, the demon, and the dragon are featured in the other part. On the one hand, being rational, she tried to convince herself that nothing can be changed, and she must move on; it happens. On the other hand, she is overwhelmed with rage, anger, and aggression. Another double-headed dragon can be seen behind the mask in its shadow. The scene validates resentment. Analyzing it, Anna was able to talk about her resentment towards her husband, his family and friends, his new partner, and even against her son. It gave her great relief.

The last mask in this trauma survival story is the self-portrait (Figure 25.4). Anna preferred modeling sand to the sand tray. While we were talking about her emotional state and last week's events, Anna kept rolling modeling sand around her finger, creating a sharp cone-shaped miniature, then removing it from the finger and placing it on the desk. She did it again and again while we were talking, until the desk was half-covered with miniatures. Afterwards, Anna used the remaining sand to make her own portrait in response to my question, "how have you changed during the therapy and what kind of person have you become." Anna responded:

> I can look back and reminisce about good moments we had with my husband. No one can take that away from me; it is my past, and I have good memories. If previously I felt like everything was killed or frozen, now my emotions are back. I am coming back to life.

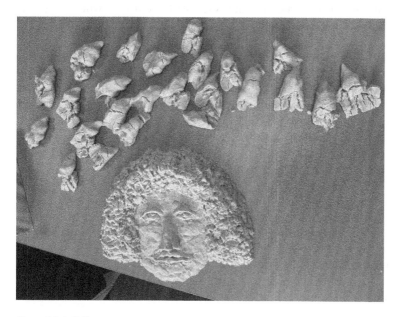

Figure 25.4 Self-portrait.

Photograph by the author.

Anna worked very carefully. It was important for her to show the structure of her hair, and she spent a fair amount of time on it, telling how it had grown in the meantime. Completing the hair, she proceeded with making the eyes, the nose, and finally the mouth. Anna did like the result. When we discussed the sequence, she acknowledged that, still, she was not able to share everything and speak out, and therefore, the mouth was the last to appear. However, she started to notice more details and observe her inner world. Watching the self-portrait and figurines described above, I reminded her of the mask of Gorgon Medusa. By working with the masks and other images, she was able to get rid of the snakes, broke Medusa's spell, and turn it back into human.

Conclusion

Throughout the sandplay sessions, Anna chose masks and figurines that represented her feelings of betrayal and came to terms with the loss of her marriage and future expectations.

The masks became survival milestones or layers that helped her to work through the crisis and breakdown of her marriage, pain of betrayal, and loss of a future she had planned. Layer by layer, they opened unconscious feelings and thoughts. Doing so, Anna went through the process of removing masks that covered her true face and was able to return to who she was at her core. Analyzing her therapy route, Anna said:

> In such a difficult situation, I lost myself. I was lost as a mother, as a woman, as a friend. I did not want to see anyone, and I felt that my life was over. I could not and would not live without my husband. At the same time, I was overwhelmed with anger and resentment that I could smash everything around myself. But I was out of energy. Here, together with you, I was building myself up from pieces. As if all your figurines are parts of myself, and I was putting those pieces together. And probably there are more parts to be put back.

No doubt, we wear different masks in our lives. Some of them limit us and do not allow us to go beyond our functions, some emerge in times of crisis or in post-traumatic periods. Masks can protect our psyche, but they can capture us by their content and deprive us of our true faces. Using various masks in sandplay therapy, we can enter the mask's functional field and reflect on its content, helping to resolve inner turmoil and restore balance between inner and outer reflections of self.

References

Adler, G., & Hull, R. F. C. (Eds.) (1971). *Psychological types: Collected works of C. G. Jung* (Vol. 6). Princeton University Press.

Ammann, R. (1991). *Healing and transformation in sandplay: Creative processes become visible*. Open Court Press.

Jung, C. J. (1981). *The archetypes and the collective unconscious* (R. F. C. Hull, Trans.). Princeton Press.

Kalff, D. (2003). *Sandplay: A psychotherapeutic approach to the psyche*. Temenos Press.

Rowling, J. K. (1997). *Harry Potter and the chamber of secrets*. Bloomsbury.

Chapter 26

The Use of Power Masks in Processing Grief

Hannah Sherebrin

My work with trauma and grief started in the early 1990s conducting workshops at the King's College International Death, Grief, and Bereavement Conference in London, Ontario. However, my personal experience of trauma and grief started when I was born during World War II in Europe. We were lucky enough to be able to escape in 1944 by boat to Turkey, and from there to British-governed Palestine. I certainly had developmental trauma, which was enhanced with the death of my brother in 1948 during the War of Independence, when I was seven years old. The scope of my work encompasses individual and group work with adults and youth suffering trauma and bereavement wounds. I have worked in palliative care, in home hospice, and conducted art therapy bereavement support groups for complex grief. I continue supervising art therapists working with complex trauma. I am passionate about making sure therapists recognize the importance of self-care. Teaching about vicarious trauma at an art therapy master's degree program at the University of MIT India and to art therapists in Ukraine is my way of protection of the protectors. My commitment to working in Ukraine is ongoing and includes supervising and teaching the unique work of art therapy as a first aid tool within ongoing war trauma in the entire community. Since October 7, 2023, I have been supporting and supervising art therapists who work with families and children displaced from the massacre area in Israel and the war, to safer areas.

Participants in grief groups describe their feelings of the event as shock and total collapse. The emotional burden of the trauma often destabilizes populations, creating hopelessness and helplessness, leading to what Bassel van der Kolk (2014) described as "speechless terror." For trauma survivors, there is often a suppression of emotional expression and an inability to master cognitive awareness and engage in verbal processing (Lusebrink & Hinz, 2016). Nonetheless, grieving a loss is a healthy and necessary process of accepting the death of loved ones. In most circumstances, there is no need for therapeutic intervention. However, when the loss is traumatic, sudden, or unexpected, it may result in complicated grief and even trigger

DOI: 10.4324/9781003365648-33

post traumatic stress disorder (PTSD; Sherebrin, 2002). It is even advised to have a debriefing first aid within the first 72 hours after the traumatic event (Elhart et al., 2019; Reema Harrison & Albert Wu, 2017). Originally designed for responders to traumatic events, critical incident stress debriefing (CISD) is a structured, brief intervention provided in a small group setting immediately following a crisis. It's designed to help people process the event to minimize symptoms of traumatic stress, depression, and anxiety. Critical incident debriefing consists of seven stages, and altogether, it lasts approximately three hours or less. When that does not happen, there have been cases reported where parents or close family members and friends suffered complex trauma and felt life had become meaningless. Suicidal ideations and depression were common, and people felt there was no reason to continue living after the death of a child, especially an only child, or a spouse.

Loss resulting from a violent act, whether war, terrorist activity, or natural disasters, causes an overwhelming external assault on the surviving individuals and is a traumatic event (Berberian et al., 2019; Saigh, 1984; Steele & Cox, 1986). Figley (1983) suggests that we look at the impact of such a traumatic event on individuals and families, which "due to the circumstances renders the survivors feeling an extreme sense of helplessness" (p. 6). He draws our attention to similarities in the emotional experiences of survivors of war combat, prisoners of war, hostages of terrorism, rape, or natural disasters. However, we must be cautious not to define traumatic stress exclusively from the perspective of an environmental event. Most literature acknowledges that the evaluation of a potential stressor must progress along the person/environment interaction model, taking individual coping mechanisms and pre-trauma life experiences into account (Rankin, 2003).

The saying "Misery is a tear in the fabric of life and not the fabric itself" resonates with me. Working with bereaved parents consists of mending the fabric, reweaving the remnants, creating growth, and rekindling hope. The internal anguish that underlies memory and emotion may be uncovered and managed through creativity. This provides opportunities for mastery and control not otherwise available in more traditional modes of therapeutic intervention. Creating, reorganizing, and recognising the process of change within artistic creation serves as a metaphor for the integration of losses. The act of artistic creation triggers the understanding of the possibility to change, rebuild, reshape, and create new realities.

Development of the Use of Masks

Bereavement support groups started in Israel after the Yom Kippur War of 1972 because of the large number of casualties and the demand on the Defense Ministry to provide help to bereaved parents. Support groups became an economical as well as an accepted means of treatment. The idea of creating an art therapy support group for parents whose children were killed in army conflict or terror attacks was based on the understanding that the artistic creation itself would provide a stimulus for understanding the possibility of change and lead to flexibility. Rebuilding of a new self, as well as recreating a new or different reality, leads to finding reasons and ways for a meaningful life. Creating, reorganizing, recognizing the process of change within artistic creation serves as a metaphor for the integration of losses. The act of artistic creation triggers the understanding of the possibility to change, to rebuild, to reshape, and create new realities (Czamanski-Cohen & Weihs, 2016). Art therapist Cathy Malchiodi (1992) writes, "one of the most powerful aspects of art expression in processing loss is the ability to address fear... After all, just confronting that blank paper or the untouched materials or clay can be the most courageous of acts when one is in extreme psychic pain" (p. 117).

Bassel van der Kolk (2014) notes the extreme disconnection between thought, feelings, and the body that so many people with histories of trauma and neglect experience. His conclusions are based on his own work and a wealth of other research in three main areas of study: neuroscience, which deals with how mental processes function within the brain; developmental psychopathology, concerned with how painful experiences impact the development of mind and brain; and interpersonal neurobiology, which examines how our own behavior affects the psycho-emotional and neuro-biological states of those close to us. He believes that the most important aspect of maintaining good mental health is connection to others and finding meaning and purpose in life. Although contact and connection are often terrifying to the traumatized, social support and a sense of community are the foundation upon which a healthy relationship with our own feelings and sensations is built. The art therapy support group creates a safe and welcoming environment in which people can explore their similarities and their differences. The crucial point is that trauma robs us of what Bassel van der Kolk terms *self-leadership*, the sense of having agency over ourselves and being in charge of our own experience. The path to recovery is therefore paved with the active rebuilding of that sense of self. Art is one of the roads to calm the limbic system and bring the frontal lobe back into the picture.

Power Mask – Purpose and Creation

The decision to create what I call power masks was based on the use of masks in ancient tribal rituals for rekindling courage. After working for about ten sessions on group integration and trust, on flexibility and recognizing individual patterns of grieving, and on recreating from fragmented matter, the time has come to work on resilience and growth. Different materials were used in order to increase and recognize individual resilience. Sessions were devoted to creating a group resilience puzzle based on the work of Sherebrin (2002). It also included creating from black construction paper, which I use based on my personal experience in Tamar Chazut's workshop (Art Therapist, expert in trauma – Trauma works). A group member's work with black construction paper prompted me to understand that at this stage of therapeutic intervention we need to work on individual empowerment. The work he created was a three-dimensional black paper cube; he filled it with water, commenting "one of these days it will explode" (Figure 26.1). His wife created a black paper plant with some green and red touches of color, which she stuck into the water, saying: "The water will feed the plant, it will drink the tears, and will bloom again." The renewed way of looking at the experience and the ability to express it in a new form allowed for a different perspective. Distancing

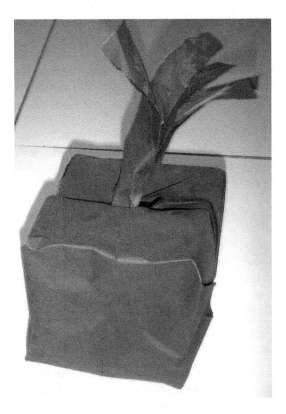

Figure 26.1 Black paper cube.
Photograph by the author.

ourselves, we can see it as well through others' eyes, and experience the pain differently.

Other emotions emerged from the pain, including anger. Anger is part of grief and trauma. It presents in various grief stages rather than being a stage itself. Therefore, if we are successful in harnessing anger, it can become a catalyst for change and for growth. Clay, as a material, lends itself to work managing anger, since hard work is required in order to make it pliable (Lusebrink & Hinz, 2016). In order to create a new stable object, clay needs to be kneaded. As we expend energy in kneading the clay, the anger can be combined into the kneading, and within the subject/object used to create a new image. Clay of course is pliable, somewhat like we are, and needs to be molded and dried for a new object to be stable and hold up the new form. Similar to clay, we learn that in order for the new creation to survive it needs to dry, rest, and eventually become permanent. This process takes time, patience, and the ability to let go.

Creating clay masks becomes a metaphor for creating ourselves as a new whole from the fragments. It was introduced at the time in which the group trusted each other and the therapy process. The time was ripe to create "masks of resilience," which the group named power masks. It expressed a new stage in the therapy process. The method I developed called for creating two masks, one of clay, the other of papier-mâché. Newspapers are crumpled into a ball the size of a head and placed on a board. Clay is rolled out and placed over the "head." Each person fashions their clay into a semblance of a face. Often, one can see the resemblance of the creator's face, which is totally unconscious. Saran Wrap (a thin plastic) is placed on the clay face, then wet papier-mâché is placed onto it in several layers in order to create the outer mask. It stays in this condition for a week. When the outer mask dries, it is pried away from the clay, and the clay mask stays as is to dry. Participants commented that the act of separating the two masks felt to them like a birthing experience. The sound that is created by prying the two masks apart is akin to the sound that can be heard with the emergence of a baby out of the birthing canal. The papier-mâché mask symbolizes an emergence of a new self, with powers of resilience and new coping skills. Paint, glue, feathers, sparkles, and found objects are all utilized to form the new mask. Each mask is different, like every person who created it.

An Example of Mask Making Effect

While working on the dried papier-mâché masks, each person concentrated on using paint, glue, bits of paper, glitter, and whatever they thought would be able to express their newfound strength to express their resilience. The silence and concentration were palpable in the room. When I circulated to make sure each person had the materials they needed, I was awed by the

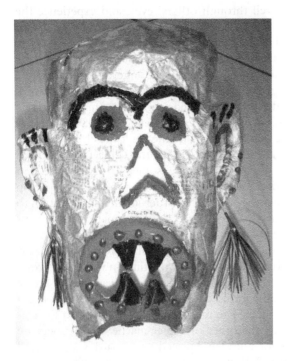

Figure 26.2 Big teeth, open mouth.
Photograph by the author.

different expressions of change in each of the participants. When they were all finished, they placed the masks on themselves, looked into a mirror, and let the masks talk. One of the masks, with big teeth and an open mouth, was created by a quiet and gentle man, who rarely spoke up in discussions (Figure 26.2). This was the first time he was able to show his anger and harness it. He found his voice. He decided to become active and tell the story of harassment and bullying in the army unit which killed his son. His wife, who created a majestic, assertive queen mask (Figure 26.3), spoke from the mirror about leading the initiative and demanding from the unit commanders to let them visit all new recruits. Anger led them to action, to express themselves and lecture the army recruits about bullying, telling them of their son's story and tragic death. Making sure they are not afraid to speak out about harassment.

Another example of change happened with the man mentioned above, who created the water cube. He was now able to create a mask which was half black and half shades of gray. He commented, when donning the mask and looking in the mirror, "I see shades on half of my face. I think I may be

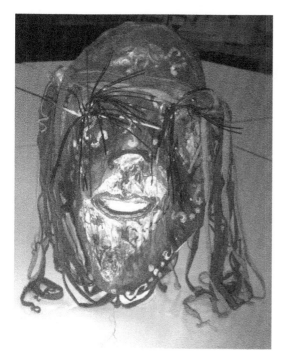

Figure 26.3 Queen mask.

Photograph by the author.

able to even use some color soon." This ability to recognize the change in the state of his reaction from passive collapse to possible movement enabled him to go back to work. His wife, the one who placed the "tree" in his cube, created a calm, dreamy mask with soothing colors and talked into the mirror about needing to show her love to the remaining two children. Each and every one of the participants was able to find ways of expression through donning the mask and speaking to the group in the mirror. The group was attentive, supporting, and embracing the way they changed. The combination of creating and being supported within the group turned out to be the key to integrating the trauma.

The clay masks are left on the shelf to dry, unpainted. The previous raw self exists unchanged and will always be there. The raw pain and the memory will always exist. Each one in the group will eventually find a place to keep the untouched clay mask in their home, garden, or wherever they feel. The place can also change with time. A place will also exist for the pain and memory, which will be integrated into the new reality of life.

The act of artistic creation leads to understanding and to the ability to discover a personal subjective reality (Fisher, 2021; Graham-Pole & Lander,

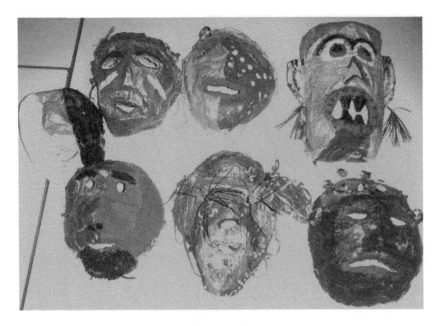

Figure 26.4 Some of the group's masks.

Photograph by the author.

2009; McNiff, 2008). Creating and donning the power masks aided the grieving parents in recognizing and embracing new roles in their lives. They found ways both to commemorate their losses and to contribute to society each in their own way (Figure 26.4).

Conclusion

With over 40 years of experience in the field of trauma and grief, I've witnessed the profound impact it has on a person's life, especially when the loss is unexpected and sudden, resulting from violence, war, terrorist activity, or natural disasters. The use of masks in art therapy can be very powerful and is used in individual, family, and group therapy. Masks can help clients integrate the loss that they have experienced and turn feelings of helplessness and hopelessness into strength. The group reenacts and creates a ritual. Through mask making, wearing the mask, and acting with the mask on, clients can rebuild the past, reshape the present, and transform their future. Mask making and using in ceremonial and healing rituals are some of the most ancient of activities. Like with all rituals, we need to be careful that we, as therapists, know when to introduce it. We also need to make sure the group trusts each other and we have the trust of the group. I accept that none of us has total control, and therefore I trust in the process to work its own magic.

References

Berberian, M., Walker, M. S., & Kaimal, G. (2019). Master my demons: Art therapy montage paintings by active-duty military service members with traumatic brain injury and post-traumatic stress. *Medical Humanities, 45*(4), 353–360. https://doi.org/10.1136/medhum-2018-01149

Czamanski-Cohen, J., & Weihs, K. L. (2016). The bodymind model: A platform for studying the mechanisms of change induced by art therapy. *The Arts in Psychotherapy, 51,* 63–71. https://doi.org/10.1016/j.aip.2016.08.006

Elhart, M., Dotson, J., & Smart, D. (2019). Psychological debriefing of hospital emergency personnel: Review of critical incident stress debriefing. *International Journal of Nursing Student Scholarship (IJNSS), 6,* 2–17. https://journalhosting.ucalgary.ca/index.php/ijnss/article/download/68395/53131

Figley, C. R. (1983). Catastrophes: An overview of family reactions. In C. R. Figley & H. I. McCubbin (Eds.), *Stress and the family* (pp. 3–20). Brunner/Mazel.

Fisher, J. (2021). *Transforming the living legacy of trauma: A workbook for survivors and therapists.* PESI Publishing & Media.

Graham-Pole, J., & Lander, D. (2009). Metaphors of loss and transition: An appreciative inquiry. *Art and Health, 1*(1), 74–88. https://doi.org/10.1080/17533010802527977

Lusebrink, V. B., & Hinz, L. D. (2016). The expressive therapies continuum as a framework in the treatment of trauma. In J. King (Ed.), *Art therapy, trauma, and neuroscience: Theoretical and practical perspectives* (pp. 42–66). Routledge.

Malchiodi, C. A. (1992). Art and loss. *Art Therapy: Journal of the American Art Therapy Association, 9*(3), 114–118. https://doi.org/10.1080/07421656.1992.10758946

McNiff, S. (2008). Art-based research. In J. G. Knowles & A. L. Cole (Eds.), *Handbook of the arts in qualitative research* (pp. 29–40). Sage.

Rankin, A. B. (2003). A task-oriented approach to art Therapy in trauma treatment. *Art Therapy: Journal of the American Art Therapy Association, 20*(3), 138–147. https://doi.org/10.1080/07421656.2003.10129570

Saigh, P. (1984). Pre- and post-invasion anxiety in Lebanon. *Behavior Therapy, 15*(2), 185–190. https://doi.org/10.1016/S0005-7894(84)80019-2

Sherebrin, H. (2002). Partners in complicated grief: National grief reactions to disasters and grassroots memorialization. In G. R. Cox, R. A. Bendiksen & R. G. Stevenson (Eds.), *Complicated grief and bereavement: Understanding and treating people experiencing loss* (pp. 241–254). Baywood Publishing Company, Inc.

Steele, K., & Cox, T. (1986). Psychological and physiological reactions to visual representations of war. *International Journal of Psychophysiology, 3*(4), 237–252. https://doi.org/10.1016/0167-8760(86)90033-4

Van der Kolk, B. A. (2014). *The body keeps the score: Brain, mind, and body in the healing of trauma.* Viking.

Chapter 27

Exploring Inner Emotions Using Masks with Children and Youth

Todd Wharton

As an art therapist working in a children's hospital with patients diagnosed with cancer, one of the keys to a successful therapeutic relationship has been allowing them to guide their own therapy. This patient population enters therapy at a time when they have been given a life-threatening diagnosis, resulting in a loss of control over their life and many new expectations and restrictions being placed upon them. Involvement in art therapy can assist in maintaining a locus of control and identity while simultaneously being able to process thoughts and emotions and learn new coping strategies related to their diagnosis and treatment.

Art Therapy and Cancer Treatment

During the early investigation and subsequent treatment phases of their journey, simply processing the cancer diagnosis itself can last well beyond the initiation of their treatment protocols. For teens especially, it has been my experience that some do more processing after completion of treatment or, when given a poor prognosis after treatment completion, have not returned favorable results. As a therapist, being aware and making allowances for youth needing to process their diagnosis when they are ready has facilitated patients getting beyond their distress and moving forward to formulate coping strategies.

Multiple times, patients old enough to understand the term "cancer" immediately report their cancer diagnosis equating to a death sentence. They often experience a significant level of grief and loss. This includes, and is not limited to, the distress caused by therapy (chemotherapy, radiation, surgery including amputation), disruptions to daily life, socializing with friends, constantly feeling unwell, unwanted physical changes, poor energy levels, hair loss, inability to participate in favored activities, impact on academic performance, and future goals. Simultaneously, parents and siblings are impacted by the diagnosis and treatment, which can make it difficult

DOI: 10.4324/9781003365648-34

to understand and support the needs of the child or youth diagnosed with cancer.

A common theme for youth undergoing treatment (chemotherapy, radiation, surgery) can include the loss of identity. One technique offered targets some of the incongruity of the internal anguish versus what the youth expresses to others. Many patients have identified feeling lost, alone, fearful, angry, isolated – truly a myriad of emotions. On the surface, they may show "good coping" or "I'm fine." Parents, friends, and others are never informed of their true inner thoughts and emotions. Some have stated they do not wish to burden their parents/caregivers any more than they already have. Others discuss the lack of understanding/empathy of important people in their lives and are given the message to simply just deal with it.

Mask Making

In working with young patients who have medical or mental health issues, the creation and processing of masks have been beneficial in allowing for identification and expression of thoughts and emotions. It can be a powerful tool in encouraging these to emerge in a safe manner within the therapeutic relationship. It should be emphasized that, due to the potential this technique can have to trigger past negative life experiences, the use of masks is recommended for those more skilled clinicians who have developed a good clinical understanding of the patients they work with and have a clear knowledge of the limits of the patient's safety boundaries. Working from a trauma-informed lens will be most beneficial for the patients in providing a safe and supportive therapeutic environment, allowing for the best clinical outcomes and, more importantly, a more positive experience for the patient. It is always best to avoid situations where well-meaning therapists/counselors who have not understood the importance of being trauma-informed have unintentionally triggered patients and either do not recognize when a patient has been triggered or know how to process the patient's unexpected emotional state, thereby creating a poor experience for the person. Mask techniques have been demonstrated to work in both individual and group settings, sometimes adapting the theme and exploratory questions to the individual participant(s).

I have incorporated two types of masks. One is a ready-made mask of pressed paper/cardboard that some manufacturers label as papier-mâché. The advantage of this type of mask is its smooth sides, which allow the patient to easily decorate and write on each side, is much less time-consuming, and works better when conducting group therapy. The other mask type uses plaster bandages applied to plastic mask molds of varying human or animal faces. The patient will line the mask with moistened plaster bandages and, once dried, they are easily removed from the mold. This mask type has the advantage of allowing more time to engage the patient in rapport-building prior to decorating and processing their mask. The disadvantage is that the inside of the mask is rough, making it difficult to decorate. The other downside to plaster masks is the limited media that can be used given the plaster's composition. Media to decorate the mask can include paint, markers, colored pencils, glitter glue, sequins, cotton balls/pompoms, stickers, beads, feathers, and fabric. Some situations may call for the use of collage or more tactile media such as clay. This technique can be adapted to the needs of the patient or availability of resources. Simple paper masks have been used impromptu by drawing and cutting out a mask shape from paper or cardstock.

Mask Making Directives

For each patient, it's different and a different process. The well-seasoned art therapist should be able to individualize the application of the mask technique. When they are well acquainted with the patient's history, the therapist can help guide them towards greater insight and expression as well as away from overwhelming themself. Using the available media, the patient is instructed to place symbols, words, and colors on the "exterior" of the mask, representing what they show to the world in a manner that best suits how they wish to portray the external self. The patient is also provided with directions to replicate a similar theme with a more genuine representation of their authentic self, which may include positive and distressing aspects, on the inner surface of the mask. The therapist is to communicate with their patient to only represent what they feel safe doing, limiting any potential to overwhelm the patient. The patient decides which side of the mask they would like to start with. For some, it may be a back-and-forth process of mask completion while for others, one side is completed prior to starting on the reverse side. Masks, in my experience, have been utilized in different and effective ways. Whatever the technique selected, it should be tailored to the patient, considering their developmental age, coping skills, resiliency, and the goals of therapy. I have utilized masks for either fictional representation or reflection/expression.

Fictional Representation

Using a mask technique which focuses on the fictional representation approach can provide the opportunity to safely allow thoughts and emotions to be expressed in a less direct manner. Through the use of fictional representation, one can direct internal thoughts and emotions onto a mask which may be a step towards identifying less recognized and/or more sensitive thoughts and emotions. Making the abstract internal experiences more concrete via the process of creating a mask opens an opportunity for greater insight. Fictional representation approaches include representing oneself as an animal, superhero, idols, cartoon, or anime character. Fictional representation tends to be used more for younger patients or those requiring a less directive approach due to vulnerability.

Implementing the fictional representation approach can involve the use of ready-made masks or creating a mask from plaster bandages and a mask mold. When selecting the plaster mold, the process of creating the mask itself can include early relationship-building discussions, introducing the purpose of the project, and beginning to explore the patient's perspective. Once the type of mask is selected or constructed, the patient is requested to complete the face or exterior of the mask by applying available media, rendering it close to how the character is typically portrayed or in a way which best represents the qualities the person likes, admires, etc. This can be achieved by placing symbols, words, colors on the face or exterior of the mask. If wanting to take the process one step further, the patient can be asked about ways they might wish to be more like the character they have created by applying media on the inner side or "interior" of the mask. More of the patient's thoughts and emotions may become uncovered, which may lead to further exploration and potential discussions regarding future goals.

Reflection/Expression

Using masks as a form of reflection/expression is typically the technique offered. However, depending on the circumstances, a projection mask may be offered initially, with a reflection/expression mask offered later in therapy. The inside can reflect inner thoughts and emotions. These can be literal or representational, symbolic, and meaningful to the individual, whatever is a fit for the patient. The outer aspect of the mask can reflect what is shown and expressed to the world, again, in concrete or abstract representational; whatever is important to the patient. Through processing the mask with the patient, they give meaning to their mask and engage in discussions of the relationship between the art, their thoughts, emotions, and their state of being. This can then lead to the identification of their concerns and issues advancing towards the development of plans for learning new coping strategies and/or informing others of their need for congruency and how best to communicate these. For others, simply being given the opportunity to spend time with the art therapist and discussing their mask and the meaning may be all they are able or choose to do.

Using the mask for reflection/expression typically includes a preliminary discussion before executing the technique. This typically involves the art therapist discussing the "masks" all people wear, being the "face" we present to the world, followed by concrete examples of what this entails. An illustrative example would be someone having a particularly difficult personal issue but maintaining a positive and/or professional demeanor while at school/work. This can lead into a general discussion about medical or mental health issues/stresses people may be experiencing while appearing to the outside world as being "all good," when internally they may be experiencing various levels of unhappiness, sadness, or distress. Through previous work with the patient, the therapist may then provide examples of past knowledge of what previous patients in similar circumstances may have been thinking and feeling, citing that there can be quite a large range of experiences and that each person's experience is uniquely their own and no two people are the same. That does not mean, however, there can't be some similarities, but that the patient is required to follow a particular path/script.

Using the reflection/expression approach with siblings of patients diagnosed with cancer has its unique perspective. Giving siblings the opportunity to create masks allows for the expression of the emotional impact of being a sibling of someone diagnosed with cancer. It has generally been the case that siblings typically do not communicate the significant impact of living with someone who has a cancer diagnosis. Certainly, it's common that younger patients tend to exhibit behavioral expressions of the disruptions. However, older patients tend not to share their experience. The mask technique gives permission for siblings to freely voice, through creative expression, their personal challenges. Offering this technique has shown itself to be a real door opener in a group setting and has generated valuable discussions of shared experiences including guilt, anger, jealousy, life disruptions, loss of attention, loss of routine, to name but a few.

In working with bereaved siblings, the use of masks using the reflective/expressive approach has been effective in providing the opportunity for siblings to process their grief. One technique is having siblings re-create memories of the brother/sister on the outside of the mask, focusing on the positive aspects of the relationship. Another similar approach involves representing the memories of the lost person on the outside while representing their grief on the inside of the mask. For some, mixed emotions are expressed representing anger, sadness, confusion, loneliness, and guilt. This technique can be a stepping stone to identifying and further processing aspects of the grief the person is experiencing. Siblings are given the message that relationships are a mixture of good and not so good, and the emotions we experience in grief are as well. For others, simply being given the opportunity to have an outlet such as creating and processing a mask to represent grief in an open and non-judgmental milieu has been reported to be a positive step in their journey. Many siblings have reported not wanting to burden parents during their time of grief to seek support, or some have feared being judged for their thoughts and feelings and elect to not express these directly. Being able to communicate to an objective person, the art therapist, allows for the safe expression of any emotions the person may be experiencing and being able to move forward with their lives. Through this support, taking it one step further, the art therapist may be able to assist siblings to communicate aspects of their grief to their caregivers.

Other Populations

Mask technique can be applied in a variety of other settings. In working with the 2SLGBTQAI community, using masks allows for the opportunity for processing one's gender identity and/or sexual orientation. In applying the reflective/expression approach, having the person use the inside of the mask as a visual representation of their authentic self can assist with identifying who they feel they are and processing the need for self-acceptance. This can be effective with gender identity and sexual orientation issues. The outside of the mask could initially be utilized to explore goal setting for gender expression, both in terms of exploring what gender expression goals one may have or creating a more concrete plan for how best to translate these goals into reality. The outside of the mask can demonstrate how they wish to represent themselves to the world, during and after social transition. This can make way for discussions regarding how best to inform others of their true self and to develop coping strategies with the responses from people in their world.

Processing the Mask

After the patient has completed the mask, the therapist can begin to process the side of the mask the patient identifies as the safest. The creative work of the patient is explored in terms of meaning and impact. Processing takes as long as required, ensuring safe boundaries are consistently maintained. For some, simply being given permission to express their authentic self through visual art may also be the first time they have reflected on the divide between their external and internal selves or acknowledged the possible distress/negative life events in a more concrete and formal manner. The therapist processes the mask until the sense of completion has occurred.

This work can be revisited in future sessions when therapeutically indicated. Insight can occur at different times throughout the course of therapy, and simply referring to the technique itself may be all that is needed. Depending on the patient's goals and changes in status or understanding, multiple masks may be completed. For others, one time may be sufficient.

In working with palliative young patients, much of the contact with the patients would have started shortly after the time of a cancer diagnosis. Thus, there would already have been an established therapeutic alliance. Knowing one has been given a terminal prognosis is devastating. Some palliation is short in duration while others may be longer. The role of the art therapist requires being in the moment for patients and working with them to set goals and support their needs. Integrating masks is different for each person. Some wish to leave their mark and create works of art which do not necessarily reflect their expressed emotions. Rather, they wish to leave their stamp, an indication they were here, a symbol of their existence. Others have used masks to process their emotions. Some may speak very little while creating their mask while others have something to say. It's about creating the opportunity for the patient to use their time in their way. Taking the cue from the patient, either during the creation of the mask or processing it afterwards, meaningful conversations can occur focusing on their life lived, memories, experiences, highlights. This may also include engaging in discussions about regrets and the grief of having a life end before expected and the impact that has on them. Some conversations are quite open about thoughts and emotions regarding their impending death, conversations the patient may not necessarily have with any other person. Masks may contain symbolic representations of what cannot be verbalized to others or to family or friends close to the person. For some, the therapist becomes an advocate or voice in communicating thoughts and wishes.

Conclusion

Throughout the years, feedback from young patients has been consistent. Many have reported that this process provides good insight, being able to more concretely understand and then express what have been their internal experiences. In addition, many have expressed relief at being given the opportunity to openly explore and express their concerns free from judgment or expectations.

Chapter 28

Masks, Grief, and the Unseen Realms

The Power of the Image

Pat B. Allen

"Art making is a way to care for loss… Grief is never entirely finished, though it may diminish and transform" (Allen, 1995, p. 138). Writing this chapter offered me the opportunity to revisit a mask I made following my father's death in 1983. I wrote about this mask in my first book *Art is a Way of Knowing* (Allen, 1995, p. 135). I was keen to delve back into the image and the mask making process for this chapter because, some years since its initial creation, that mask began to speak to me from the wall and ask for conversation and transformation. In 2008, after 25 years of existing silently, offering the simple comfort of giving form and containment to grief and memory, the image asked for more. As an artist and art therapist for over 50 years, I have hundreds of images in flat files, preserved in photos, and just existing in my memory. It is a common experience for me when discussing a clinical issue with a colleague, or seeing a theme arise in my own ongoing art practice, to recall an image from the past. When possible, I search for the image and bring it out to see what it might have to say about the current situation. If I don't have a physical image, I might enter into reverie and recall the image as best I can. Sometimes I recreate the image. I also live with many of my most significant images. The seven small oil paintings I created during my Jungian analysis early in my career have lived on the walls of either my home or my studio since the 1970s. They continue to emanate energy and information and to feel very much alive to me.

The context I offer here is scaffolded by some foundational beliefs that support and guide my creative practice. These are not theoretical, but rather have emerged from continual immersion in the process of art making and writing about what comes. These beliefs include that the image has a life of its own, it is not merely a document of a process; I can continue to be instructed by the image years after it was created; images may have multiple meanings; and images and the meanings and energies they hold can unfold and evolve over time. I believe that in the realm of the creative process there is no such thing as linear time. In addition to the common experiences of "time standing still" or "time flying by in a seeming instant" while working

DOI: 10.4324/9781003365648-35

in the studio, I suggest that the place from which images emerge is a numinous space that is both within us and greater than us. In fact, I think of it as the realm of the Divine.

I offer ideas from somatic psychology as a bridge to make these concepts perhaps more accessible to a reader who might find them strange (Gendlin, 1981). In the same way that our physical body continues to hold energy and experiences from our past, the image, which is something made by our hands, can function like an extension of the embodied self. Energy and experiences can live in an image and, like memories and experiences that live in our body, can be accessed and transformed through somatic means. In other words, no image is ever truly finished, even if it is framed and hung on a wall. Like a somatically activated memory, an imaginal need may arise and be expressed unexpectedly. This is what happened to me.

One day, the mask of my father began to call me for attention. Where months had gone by when I barely noticed the mask as I went about my daily routine, suddenly my attention was subtly snagged by the mask, and I began to see it as I might notice a change in the landscape I walk every day. This call coincided with a dream about my grandfather, my father's father. My sister had always observed that the mask of our father looked to her more like our grandfather. I had chalked that up to the fact that the last time I saw my father, he was old and may have resembled his own dad. One of the ways I responded to the mask's call was to engage in active imagination, an ancient technique described most clearly and used most frequently by Carl Jung, both in his own process as well as with his patients (Hannah, 1981). Active imagination requires us to relax our body into a state of quiet reverie, focusing on the breath and becoming quite still. In my practice, I write an intention, a sentence or two of what I am inviting into my experience.

In this case, I opened myself up to the spirit of my grandfather as well as to the spirit of the mask itself, since the dream I had the previous night was the starting point of the call. In the state of active imagination, I began a dialogue, asking my grandfather why he had come. He conveyed to me that he was stuck on his soul's journey. He mentioned seeking forgiveness for acts he had committed while alive, including harming my cousin when she was a child and an attempt at inappropriate touching of my sister. I was aware of these claims and had heard family stories on this topic. I told him I was unable to grant him any forgiveness as these were not my experiences. He then became belligerent and claimed he wasn't at fault, that the girls had initiated what occurred. I firmly rejected this idea and the conversation ended. Over the course of subsequent encounters with the mask itself over several months, the piece asked to be repainted several different times. The voice asking for repainting was not the voice of my grandfather but rather the voice of the mask itself. Each time I repainted the mask, something different was revealed. This layering served to unveil a new reality rather than to conceal something.

The first time (see Figure 28.1), I was called to simply apply a coat of gesso. Where the original mask appeared to have eyes closed or possibly looking inward, once repainted in the all-white gesso, I clearly discerned open eyes. This was quite a surprise. It also appeared much more to resemble my dad.

I lived with the mask in this form for a while and continued in active imagination with a spirit that felt like my father. He also had regrets to get off his chest. He conveyed great anguish about past events, his father's actions, and any harm that he himself had contributed through lack of awareness. I witnessed the mask and repainted it once again, this time in shades of black, white, and red. I felt the complexity of my father's experience. The sense of tangled threads unravelling was very powerful, as well as the feeling of some generational patterns being released. Eventually, over a period of several weeks of living with the mask in this state, something

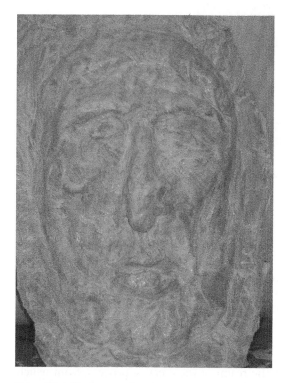

Figure 28.1 Mask painted with gesso.
Photograph by the author.

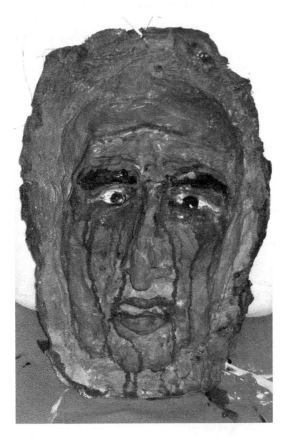

Figure 28.2 Mask painted black, white, and red.

Photograph by the author.

shifted. I experienced a sense of peace and forgiveness for both my father and grandfather. I also felt that I was being given a window into aspects of what art making can accomplish in the realm of transformative ancestral healing, that we can in fact heal our ancestors through our work in the present. This work unfolded over months at the pace dictated by the images. I made no alterations in the form of the mask except for painting and repainting (Figure 28.2). I still find it eerie that the eyes which seemed closed or inward for 25 years were now open, for the first time. I have often had this experience in the realm of the creative process, from which the image originates, there is no linear time; past, present, and future exist simultaneously.

The sense of relational connection to the spirits of those on the other side of the veil and those between worlds, as well as to the mask itself, feels extraordinarily powerful to me as well. I have no doubt that my circumstances of living in a place surrounded by mountains, trees, and solitude, as well as ample time for these experiences to unfold, contributed to this work happening. Additionally, decades of experience in art making, living with and witnessing images, and the lifelong study of the work of Carl Jung, provided me with grounding to tolerate strange experiences that would be unlikely to occur in a usual art therapy setting where time and space are limited, goals are set rationally, and a particular outcome is sought.

Figure 28.3 offers the version of the mask as it now exists. While writing this chapter, the mask asked for another repainting, this time of the unfinished edge that surrounds the face. The edge had been a greyish color, and now the mask wanted gold. When I use metallic gold in art making, I usually paint a layer of red first. The red provides warmth and depth to the gold, and I did that here. The feeling now is of a halo. While I am open to

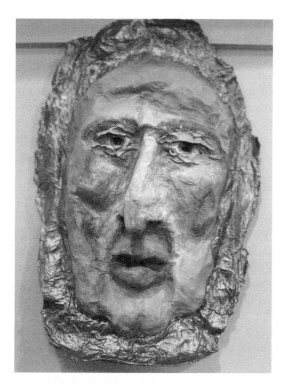

Figure 28.3 Mask outlined in gold.

Photograph by the author.

making further changes if the mask requires them, it seems to be at rest for the moment. The sense I now have is that the face is circled by a halo, a feature of art that usually denotes a divine or spiritual aspect. I feel a sense of having aided my relatives on their souls' journeys and helped them to join the divine realm.[1]

I find support for the importance of ongoing engagement with an art piece over time in the el duende work of art therapist Abbe Miller (2020). In the el duende painting process, the artist works on the same canvas multiple times with pauses in between of not painting. The artist simply lives with the image as it unfolds. It is common for images to appear in the painting process and to be layered over with other images multiple times as the process continues. Rather than an act of covering or obscuring, layering reveals new meanings as images arrive via the portal opened by the artist's intention to invite them onto the canvas and into awareness. During the process of writing this piece, I found myself experiencing resistance to engaging with the subject of the mask and what was required for me to make the experience understandable to others. Yet, I felt a gentle insistence by the image to share this work. When I tried doing other creative tasks, it felt as if a cloud had moved into my internal landscape and my energy waned. As I often do when feeling blocked, I made an intention to see why this resistance was occurring. I made a quick scribble and wrote a simple witness and was directed firmly to the mask and writing this chapter (Allen, 2005).

I recently turned 70 years of age and have been contemplating the meaning of this phase of life, particularly regarding art therapy and my creative process. As is common towards the end of a long career, I have been reviewing themes, assessing my contributions, and discerning how much energy I have to do more. *Art is a Way of Knowing* (1995) marked a major shift from my early clinical practice to considering and defining for myself what art therapy meant to me. In addition to the book, I co-founded the Open Studio Project and spent many years exploring which aspects of art therapy mattered to me and which I would choose to discard. I had by that time more than a decade of experience as an art therapist in clinical settings including a psychiatric unit, substance abuse, juvenile justice, physical rehabilitation, community mental health center, and private practice. And while the art therapy field sought recognition and credentialing in clinical mental health service delivery as its major focus, I deepened my involvement in art making and questioned the role of the therapist. I was called to develop an alternative model called the open studio process (OSP), in which spirituality and art are central, and clinical considerations are generally entirely set aside.

The OSP model (Allen, 2005) emphasizes the role of the artist and seeks to activate this aspect of self in all who participate together in a studio setting. Through the process of setting an intention, each person assumes sovereignty over their own creative process. Art for me is a means to connect to something greater and beyond myself and to have an intimate relationship with this life force, which I call the creative source. While the nature of the OSP can be experienced as therapeutic, it does not rely on the presence of a therapist. Instead, the relationship that is created is with one's deepest self. A significant aspect of OSP is the writing practice that accompanies art making. Margaret Naumburg, one of art therapy's founders and my mentor, recommended a journaling practice after making art in which the page is divided so that thoughts, feelings, and relevant dreams can be recorded over time.[2] I have named this witness writing, which describes the process of writing a response to art that is created. This allows each person to bring their cognitive and thinking mind into alignment with the intuitive self-aspect from which the image arises, allowing one to be a witness to the art making. The artist and witness capacities of self, working together, can supply many of the experiences that are sought after in therapy as well as in spiritual practices. I certainly acknowledge that having another person in the role of therapist can be beneficial. However, the autonomous and self-directed aspects of OSP can open avenues that might not be available in traditional art therapy due to constraints of systems in which art therapy is practiced.

The mask work represents an intersection of healing soul work as well as an acknowledgment of a realm beyond what we see in ordinary reality. Like many art therapists, I have been touched by the upheaval in culture, consciousness, and politics in the last decade, exacerbated by the collective experience of COVID-19. The current iteration echoes and deepens what was occurring in the 1970s when I entered the field of art therapy. I believe we are being collectively called to expand our consciousness about many things, including harm done by our forebears and our own participation in continuing systems of oppression. The idea of generational trauma and collective ancestral healing is very alive for me (Menakem, 2017). The mask feels like an example of such work on the personal level, and I believe we can gather to support such work collectively. The image can be a portal to meaning, but whose messages are revealed only when consciously invited and engaged, and when we can support one another in doing so with care and understanding.

Summary

Art making and art therapy have enormous untapped potential to enable us to engage the unseen realm of energy, soul, and spirit. In the infinite realm of the creative process, there are resources to ease, heal, and transform patterns of harm in families and in cultures. Art making is a powerful means to reweave ourselves into new ways of being with one another and with the natural world, and to unravel and understand ancestral stories of suffering and wisdom. I hope this chapter offers an expanded view of the boundaries of art therapy and offers an invitation to others to explore the unseen realms in the service of healing and expanding our conscious awareness both personally and collectively.

Notes

1 To see the images of this chapter in color, visit www.patballen.com.
2 Although I have never come across a mention of this practice in Naumburg's writings, it was one that she recommended to me during the time she mentored me in art therapy and which has become a lifelong practice.

References

Allen, P. B. (1995). *Art is a way of knowing: A guide to self-knowledge and spiritual fulfillment through creativity.* Shambhala Publications.
Allen, P. B. (2005). *Art is a spiritual path: Engaging the sacred through the practice of art and writing.* Shambhala Publications.
Gendlin, E. T. (1981). *Focusing.* Bantam Books.
Hannah, B. (1981). *Encounters with the soul: Active imagination in the life and work of C. G. Jung.* Sigo Press.
Menakem, R. (2017). *My grandmother's hands: Racialized trauma and the pathway to mending our hearts and bodies.* Central Recovery Press.
Miller, A. (2020). *One-canvas method: Art making that transforms on one surface over a sustained period of time* [Doctoral Dissertation, Lesley University]. DigitalCommons@ Lesley. https://digitalcommons.lesley.edu/expressive_dissertations/94/

Index

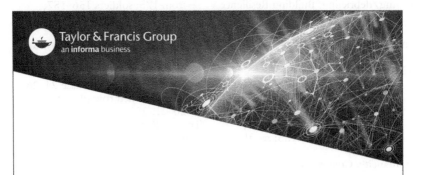

For Product Safety Concerns and Information please contact our EU representative GPSR@taylorandfrancis.com Taylor & Francis Verlag GmbH, Kaufingerstraße 24, 80331 München, Germany

Printed and bound by CPI Group (UK) Ltd, Croydon, CR0 4YY

08/06/2025

01897006-0003